Risking Life for Death
Lesson for the Living from the Autopsy Table

Risking Life for Death

*Lesson for the Living
from the Autopsy Table*

RYAN BLUMENTHAL

Jonathan Ball Publishers
Johannesburg • Cape Town

© Text: Ryan Blumenthal (2023)
© Cover image: iStock/fergregory
© Published edition: Jonathan Ball Publishers (2023)

Originally published in South Africa in 2023 by
JONATHAN BALL PUBLISHERS
A division of Media24 (Pty) Ltd
PO Box 33977
Jeppestown
2043

ISBN 978-1-77619-268-7
ebook ISBN 978-1-77619-269-4

www.jonathanball.co.za
www.twitter.com/JonathanBallPub
www.facebook.com/JonathanBallPublishers

Cover by Marius Roux
Edited by Carol-Ann Davids
Proofread by Paul Wise
Design and typesetting by Nazli Jacobs
Printed and bound by CTP Printers, Cape Town
Set in Bookman

To all those harmed, injured or killed as a result of a crime, accident or other event or action.

Contents

Preface

Since the publication of my first book, *Autopsy: Life in the Trenches with a Forensic Pathologist*, people have sent me long messages about how the book affected them. There came a flood of Facebook friendship requests, I received countless selfies on Instagram of strangers holding my book – one of these from someone in a maximum-security prison whose picture had been taken while he was in full prison uniform, with his handcuffs on, holding my book. How he managed this is beyond me. Mothers wanting career advice for their kids began contacting me. Pensioners wanted to meet me for coffee. (The youngest person claiming to have read my book was seven years old, while the oldest was 96.)

People that I would never normally have access to were suddenly trying to connect with me. Apparently, I was the only one who could solve some or other specific forensic case. One Saturday at midnight, just as I was about to retire to bed, I got a phone call from Cape Town about a suspected food poisoning case: the person was worried about a salad they had eaten. Where could they submit the salad for forensic analysis? Of course, how could I assist, when Cape Town is not even my jurisdiction?

I had a stalker (you never get the stalker you want in life): It started with gifts from an unknown admirer who had read my book and escalated from there, as these things typically do – but, luckily, the entire debacle ended amicably. Then *Autopsy* went international, and my life really changed. At the time of writing, I had received countless questions and comments from as far afield as Marion Island – a very remote island in the subantarctic Indian Ocean. (Yes, a courier company delivers books to Marion Island.) I am thrilled that my book resonated with so many people and has travelled so far.

This book, my second, expands on the lessons for the living that can be gleaned from the autopsy table. I wrote it because I feel I have a moral obligation to serve my immediate community as well as the greater community of humankind. There remains so much injustice in this world, and forensic pathology is not some sideshow but rather, I believe, plays a central role. I also wrote it because I have been feeling somewhat dissatisfied of late, and unable to tolerate the situation. So, yes, my battle is also personal.

I hope that some of the ideas in this book may resonate with you and contribute to your well-being.

Beyond that, this book will teach you how to notice the smallest of details – how to *really* notice. For example, did you know that the strength of a handshake may tell you about someone's health? Myotonic dystrophy is an inherited disorder that typically involves progressive muscle wasting and weakness. Clinical presentation of this disease is characterised by muscle weakness, cataracts, infertility (in males) and cardiac conduction defects. And so, when someone who has been diagnosed with myotonic dystrophy shakes hands, there may be a delay in relaxation of the thumb.[1] Noticing how someone releases your hand within the first few moments after a handshake may tell you a great deal.

Forensic pathology is a field of tremendous scope and breadth. In this book, I share how forensic pathologists think and solve problems and apply basic principles. I explain the first principle that underpins forensic pathology: Locard's Exchange Principle, or Contact Theory. This book seeks to be a master class in this one singular forensic technique.

Collecting all this data in a book has been like having had a thousand puzzle pieces in a box. Until you put the pieces together, you really have no idea what the final picture will look like. And now, at long last, after years of rearranging those puzzle pieces, they finally make sense, and it is my duty, and honour, to show you the importance of each puzzle piece and the view from overhead.

Please note that where the pronoun 'he' is used in the book, it is intended that the word 'she' is equally applicable – or 'they' – unless obviously inappropriate from the context. In writing this book, I have tried to be impartial and equally sympathetic to both sides (because there are always two sides).

Finally, on a completely different note, I always have plants in my office so that I can be surrounded by life, especially after spending my days surrounded by death.

Ryan Blumenthal

1

Solving puzzles

'Is there a doctor on board?' I was flying from Cape Town to Johannesburg.

The voice of the flight attendant sounded urgent. Immediately I shrank in my chair. I was sitting in a passenger seat at the front of the plane, with another 150 people on board. I am a forensic pathologist and had last seen a living patient in 2001. It was almost two decades since I'd last examined or treated a living human being, and so I was naturally hesitant to respond. At the time of the incident, I certainly didn't look like a forensic pathologist: I was wearing my comfortable travel clothing and sipping a glass of white wine, with my mind focused on other things.

'Is there a doctor on board?' the voice of the flight attendant sounded increasingly frantic.

It would be illegal for me, as a forensic pathologist, to practise clinical medicine given that this is against the rules and regulations of the Health Professions Council of South Africa. And so I listened to the flight attendant calling out as I continued to sip my wine: 'Please identify yourself if you have any medical training. We really have an emergency here.' Eish, I thought to myself, no one is putting their hand up! Reluctantly, I raised my hand and at once the flight attendant came running towards me.

'Please, doctor, we really need your help.'

'I am a forensic pathologist, a doctor of the dead. I haven't examined or treated a living patient in over twenty years. I do have some medical background knowledge, though, so if there really is no one else on board who can help, then I will see what I can do.'

'Please doctor, there really is no one else who can help!' she said pleadingly, her face flushed and deadly serious.

I got up from my seat and walked to the back of the plane. All the other passengers seemed to be watching and staring at my every move. I knew that I didn't look the part. What was going through my mind at the time was: what happens if this is a heart attack or stroke patient? What if this is a drug mule? If I opened the aeroplane's medical kit, then surely it would lead to much homework and many forms to complete. And what if the patient, tragically, were to die in my hands?

At the back of the plane, lying on the floor, was a 60-year-old female with a silver space blanket covering her body. She had an oxygen mask over her face. The woman looked diaphoretic (the medical term used to describe excessive, abnormal sweating in relation to environment or activity level).

I turned to the flight attendant. 'Please bring her some sugar water or a glass of Coca-Cola, and then bring me her overhead carry-on bag. I want to see what's inside it. I might find some pills or a clue, something that can alert me as to what's wrong with her and help with my diagnosis.'

The 60-year-old woman managed a sip or two of the sugar water and I saw that she was slowly on the mend. Phew, I thought to myself. Lucky for her (and also lucky for me).

This was probably a hypoglycaemia attack – low blood sugar – or something like that. Right at that moment the flight attendant arrived with the patient's hand luggage. I opened it . . . and guess what I found inside her bag. Drugs? No. Medicines? No. Strange devices? No.

Tucked in between her purse and her lipstick was the erotic romance novel *Fifty Shades of Grey*, by EL James. In summary, the novel follows the deepening relationship between college graduate Anastasia Steele and young business magnate Christian Grey, and is notable for its sexually explicit scenes featuring elements of sexual practices involving BDSM (standing for combinations of bondage and discipline, dominance and submission, and sadism and masochism). The bookmark was wedged between pages four and five.

'Lady . . .' I began. Her eyes were now fully open and alert as she sat upright, looking rather spritelier than minutes earlier, and decidedly less diaphoretic. 'Perhaps you should only read one page per day.'

Both the recovering woman and the flight attendant burst into laughter at this. She made a complete recovery as I sat and monitored her for the duration of the flight back to Johannesburg, my hand resting on her wrist pulse. The situation could have been worse. Much worse.

I can tell a lot of what is happening in the world from noticing what is happening on my autopsy table. I can tell if a new gang has moved into the neighbourhood. I can tell if there is a new or emergent drug or disease, and I can even get a good sense of the health (physical, mental and psychological) of the nation without necessarily having to venture out of doors. Forensic pathologists may not be physically on the streets, yet we still have a relatively good idea of what is happening. I am fascinated to know what's going on in the world by seeing it from the perspective of what's happening in the mortuary.

When I examine a body, I can tell if a deceased person was a smoker, and whether they have been in the presence of smokers recently, thanks to the difficulty of removing the smell of second-hand smoke from clothing and hair. Also, chronic smokers generally have nicotine stains on their fingers, inelastic skin and wrinkles. Their facial skin loses its lustre and they often have lung pathology. Illicit drug users also tend to have signs of the pathology of chronic drug abuse on their bodies.

I can tell if a deceased person was near fried foods or a braai (barbecue): the smallest droplets of fried or barbecued food, or of aerosolised oils, can attach themselves to spectacles, clothing and hair, proving that they were in close proximity. I am able to deduce if someone was probably a tik addict or a cannabis abuser.

I notice these things every day – and, as with the diaphoretic woman on the plane, noticing the smallest details may help one better understand a situation, providing an advantage. Noticing requires excellent eyesight, but *really* noticing requires excellence in applying all one's senses, so as to apprehend sounds, textures and odours too.

If you are reading this book, I assume you too want to notice the smallest of details, details to which the average onlooker may be oblivious. It is my desire to share one of the basic forensic principles with you, which will help you develop your forensic cognitive toolkit. You will have an extra weapon to help you critically assess and diagnose certain situations, or when you encounter information that requires critical review, like when you read something on Facebook, Instagram or WhatsApp: you will be able to interrogate it before simply forwarding it to all your friends and relatives.

It was a forensic pathologist who first determined that car power windows could be lethal when he reported the case of a 26-month-old girl who had been asphyxiated by just such a window. Gary Simmons, a forensic pathologist, was the first to highlight this previously unrecognised hazard. Now, most car power windows have a cut-out safety mechanism that stops the window closing if part of a body is stuck in it.[1]

This, indeed, is the ultimate purpose of science: based on systematic methodology, we observe, we learn and we understand the natural and social world we find ourselves in, so that this world can be made a better place for all of us.

Please note, I will not be making medical doctors or forensic pathologists of you. I will merely be sharing with you how forensic pathologists and medical detectives think. In a world where we are bombarded with information, it is my desire to help you navigate potential minefields.

First, a little more about me.

My grandmother Freda was one of the first female butchers in South Africa. One of my earliest recollections is of her carrying an animal carcass on her back. She was a tough old woman. Freda's husband was Sam Blumenthal, an actuary and, apparently, quite a bright guy. Sadly, Sam passed away when I was 17 months old and so I never got to know him. No matter, their genes fused and melded and two generations later, I arrived. I have the genetic material of a butcher *and* that of an actuary. As a forensic pathologist, I am therefore a thinking man's butcher!

Forensic medicine fascinated me from the start. I knew I wanted to be a forensic pathologist from my fourth year in medicine, when I was first exposed to the field. Forensic pathology is all about problem-solving. I love puzzles and my hobby has always been sleight-of-hand magic. In its purest form, forensic pathology is practical puzzle-solving. I was also drawn to the fact that forensic pathology is about the truth. I simply wanted to solve mysteries and, most of all, I wanted to catch bad guys.

I am grateful to have been trained by some of the discipline's leading mentors. I have had several mentors in my life (and I believe that the sign of a good leader isn't how many followers you have, but how many leaders you create). I am also extremely fortunate to have trained and spent my entire forensic pathology career, since I began my studies in this field, at a centre of excellence. I feel privileged to have nearly all the pathology disciplines housed in the same building, a practical disposition that greatly facilitates personal and professional interactions between the disciplines. Autopsies have consumed most of my adult life. I have spent more time in the autopsy suite than in almost any other pursuit. Despite my constant exposure to death and dying, dealing with decomposing bodies, and earning a fraction of what my colleagues in clinical medicine earn, I have never been put off my profession, and I have always viewed these other factors as mere technicalities. And yet I confess that some days I do not feel like performing autopsies. It may be a decomposing body, a multiple shooting case, a mob assault case, a rape-homicide case, an abandoned foetus, or a complicated anaesthetic-procedure-related death. There are times when you are so fatigued that the only thing keeping you going is your disciplined training, your basic principles, your team, your systemic methodology and the reasons you went into this field in the first place. It is a dirty job that requires the ultimate in stamina and professionalism every day, no matter how you feel. Yet the feeling I get after completing an entire medico-legal examination – and discovering the ultimate truth – far outweighs all the negatives.

If you deal with death and tragedy every day, one of the greatest challenges is to maintain a positive and optimistic attitude to self and society. I have never turned down an opportunity to talk about forensic pathology. It is a wonderful chance to share forensic insights because I believe the dead have so much to teach the living. As forensic pathologists, we are independent: we do not serve any political party and everyone benefits from our service, irrespective of whether they be left-wing or right-wing, independent, conservative or liberal.

I believe that no one is more important than anyone else in society. Cashiers, garbage collectors and hamburger-flippers all play an important role in society and keep the world turning. Forensic pathologists are but a small cog in the large wheel that keeps the machine of the world moving. Forensic pathologists know that no one is literally 'holier than thou' because we have seen plenty of leaders and holy people die in depraved circumstances. In fact, we once found a religious leader dead in a house of ill repute. After a member of the police carelessly let slip this fact to the deceased's wife, the woman was so incensed she furiously said: 'He must now bury himself!' before she stormed off, leaving us with the unenviable task of managing the delicate matter of the religious man's funeral.

Being a forensic pathologist demands humility. I have seen children die too soon and those suffering die too late. For some life is too short and for others, too long. So many these days are living longer than expected, and often there isn't enough money to cover their medical treatment or their living expenses. (I have seen people who were financially secure for most of their working lives spend their final years as paupers.) Even if you have it all, you still have to maintain it all. I have learned that life is brutal, no matter who you are, and so working as a forensic pathologist requires a degree of introspection.

I often think about friends and colleagues who studied and worked with me. Some dropped out of medicine, some were faced with terrible tragedy, some were murdered. There were cases of substance abuse and mental health disorders, while others tragically took their own lives.

One of my dear friends, Dr Cival Mills, became a quadriplegic after a car accident. Mills wrote about his life in a book published in 2010, *This Too Will Pass*.[2] Mills fell asleep at the wheel of his car after a long shift at the hospital where he was working as an intern, sustaining an unstable neck fracture. He was only 26 years old at the time and was confined to a wheelchair. Despite the accident and suffering a stroke years later, Mills refused to think of himself as being disabled, but rather saw himself as merely somewhat more challenged than other people. He took a 'never feel sorry for yourself' attitude. Dr Cival Mills died on Friday, 3 April 2015. His death was considered an unnatural death, and he ended up having a forensic autopsy at our medico-legal facility. It broke my heart.

Forensic pathologists must, as a matter of course, do a conceptual crash test of what we think we are going to find before beginning with an actual autopsy. We should predict what we believe we will encounter inside the body before cutting it open, and never just dive in, because we simply do not know what we might find. After all, there have been cases of live bombs packed inside a deceased's body, or cocked and loaded weapons concealed somewhere about the person, or uncapped needles secreted in the pockets. Even deadly animals and insects have turned up during autopsies. Do read the story of the scuba diver who was found with a dead scorpionfish in his wetsuit in my first book, *Autopsy*.

That is why, at the outset, a scene examination must be performed and a meticulous case history made.

Please note that an autopsy and a post-mortem are not the same thing. A post-mortem is the examination of a dead body to determine the cause of death, which may entail external examination of the body after death, while an autopsy is a post-mortem examination to discover the cause of death or the extent of disease, which may entail dissection of the body after death. The difference between a post-mortem and an autopsy is therefore *dissection*. The term 'post-mortem examination' is a common alternative. Unfortunately, it suffers from a lack of precision about the extent of the examination, for in some countries many bodies are disposed of after external examination (termed a 'viewing') without dissection.[3]

The first autopsy I attended in my facility as a junior forensic pathologist was quite overwhelming. While some of the finer details of the case elude me right now, what I can clearly recall is that it was a sensory overload. The woman, who was a true beauty, had flown to Mauritius with her new husband and died suddenly and unexpectedly while having breakfast one morning. What makes this story even more remarkable is that there was a medical conference at the same hotel at that exact time. Almost all the guests having breakfast were qualified medical practitioners, yet none succeeded in resuscitating her. Her autopsy was performed in Mauritius and another was performed in South Africa. I attended the repeat autopsy.

The cause of death of the young bride was stated as saddle pulmonary embolism: a large blood clot had straddled the bifurcation of her pulmonary trunk. This condition is typically and immediately fatal.

I have seen many cases of pulmonary thromboembolism over the years. It typically looks like a little coiled black octopus straddling the pulmonary artery bifurcation. The blood clot has alternating black and grey areas within it. The black and grey areas (lines of Zahn) originate from enmeshed red blood cells, fibrin and platelets, which reflect the area of origin in the lumen of a vein in the pelvis or legs, typically an area of sluggish blood flow. Pulmonary thromboembolism is due to a blood clot (deep vein thrombosis) that travels to the lungs from the deep veins in the legs or from veins in other parts of the body, such as the pelvis.

Before her honeymoon, the young woman had started taking oral contraceptive pills, which had likely increased her risk of blood clotting. She sat still on an aeroplane for quite a few hours, which also increased her risk factors for deep venous thrombosis. (Immobilisation may lead to venous thrombosis in the lower extremities. Portions of this stasis thrombus may break away, travel through the venous circulation and lodge in the branches of the pulmonary artery.) The oral contraceptives and 'economy class syndrome' – which can also happen in first class, by the way – had a deadly impact on the young woman.

Pulmonary emboli may vary in size from large saddle emboli, which can obstruct the bifurcation of the pulmonary artery and produce sudden death, such as in this case, to less clinically significant smaller emboli, which can obstruct branches of the pulmonary artery and lead to pulmonary infarctions, which are wedge-shaped and located just beneath the pleura. People who are at risk for pulmonary embolism are typically those who have been inactive or immobile for long periods or people who have certain inherited conditions, such as blood clotting disorders.

Other risk factors include surgery and broken leg bones, while people who have cancer, smoke or are pregnant have also been associated with pulmonary embolism. Background cardiovascular diseases such as stroke, paralysis, chronic heart disease and high blood pressure have also been cited as increasing the risk for deep venous thrombosis and pulmonary embolism. A saddle pulmonary embolism is probably one of the quickest deaths. The cause of death is acute right-sided heart failure, a condition known as acute cor pulmonale. It is almost as if the right side of your heart were pumping against a brick wall.

These many years later, I wonder: if it were not for the woman's beauty, or the fact that her death happened on her honeymoon – or perhaps the fact that it was my first autopsy, or that it happened in the middle of a medical conference – would I still remember this case? Having performed thousands of forensic autopsies, I often think: what if the pulmonary embolism had happened to someone else? Would it have affected me as much and would I still remember?

It is a fact that I simply cannot forget . . .

2

Locard's Exchange Principle

A few years ago, a man was found dead on the floor of his kitchen in the east of my jurisdiction. We could see that there had been no breaking or entering. We knew that the man lived alone and that his family only discovered his inert body when they were unable to get hold of him. I was called in because this was considered a mysterious death, an unexplained death, or a SUDA – the sudden unexpected death of an adult.

I arrived on the scene in the evening and began by carefully observing the environment and noticing what often might seem irrelevant: at the scene there was an open jar of peanut butter (smooth, not crunchy) and there was a peanut-butter-stained spoon near the body. What was going through my mind at the time was the following: could this be an anaphylactic death (death resulting from an acute allergic reaction to an antigen, such as a bee-sting, to which the body has become hypersensitive)? Was he allergic to peanuts? And yet, at the same time, I was thinking: if he were allergic to peanuts, then surely he would have known about it? Why would he then be eating peanut butter?

The mystery could only be solved at autopsy, and it was at this point that I found what could only be described as a huge glob of peanut butter obstructing the upper pharynx, posterior palate and inner larynx of the deceased. It looked like complete upper airway obstruction due to peanut butter. There were no signs of anaphylaxis. No urticaria on the skin. Nothing else could explain or have contributed to his death. There were some signs suggestive of an asphyxia-type death at autopsy.

I never formally published this case, because over the years I have performed autopsies on a couple of people who have choked to death on other food material, such as steak, brown bread and sushi, for example. Choking refers to blockage of the internal airways, and death is typically the result of pure hypoxia – an absence of enough oxygen in the tissues to sustain bodily functions. This man apparently choked to death on smooth peanut butter, a fact that I still have some difficulty accepting. Who would have thought that this was even possible? Yet the evidence was undeniable.

What steps did I, as the forensic pathologist, take to arrive at a diagnosis on this case (and, indeed, all my cases)? What informs forensic pathologists even before we perform the actual autopsy? What is in the cognitive toolkit that we use?

The First Principle is the bedrock of modern forensics. Everyone's favourite detective uses this principle, without naming it:. Sherlock Holmes, Hercule Poirot, Philip Marlowe, Miss Marple, Jessica Fletcher, Thomas Magnum, Nancy Drew, Columbo, Patrick Jane, Adrian Monk and even Tintin have all at one point or another used this singular forensic principle. It is called Locard's Exchange Principle.

Dr Edmond Locard was a pioneer of forensic science. It was he who formulated the basic principle of forensic science: 'With contact between two items, there will be an exchange,' or, stated another way, 'Every contact leaves a trace.'

Born in Saint-Chamond in France on 13 November 1877, Locard studied medicine in Lyon. He went on to publish more than 40 works, the most famous being his seven-volume series *Traité de Criminalistique* (*Treatise on Criminalistics*). Locard began his professional career by assisting Alexandre Lacassagne, a criminologist, physician and professor. In 1910 the Lyon Police Department granted Locard the opportunity to create, in a previously unused attic, the first crime investigation laboratory, where he could analyse evidence from crime scenes.

Locard worked as a medical examiner during World War I and managed to identify cause and location of death by analysing stains or dirt left on soldiers' uniforms. He developed multiple methods of forensic analysis, and several police laboratories were created based on the work that he did.

Locard's Exchange Principle holds, in essence, that the perpetrator of a crime will bring something into the crime scene and will leave with something from it, and that both of these can be used as forensic evidence.

It can be the smallest of things that ensures a criminal is caught. A classic example of Locard's Exchange Principle is where fragmentary, or trace, evidence is left at, or taken from, a crime scene: where there is contact between two surfaces, such as shoes and the soil, or when fibres are left behind.

Let me give you a personal example. Many years ago, a medical colleague and friend gave me, as a gift, three rare quails. I carefully placed the quails in my small back garden and immediately set off to the pet store to buy a cage. When I returned, all three of my quails lay dead! And this, only a few hours after I had received them. Within moments of finding my murdered quails, I knocked at my neighbour's door.

'Your cat just killed my quails!' I said, very upset.

'I am sorry to hear about your quails,' my neighbour replied, 'but it is in the nature of cats to roam . . . and besides, how do you know it was *my* cat who killed your quails?'

'Lady,' I responded, 'I am a forensic pathologist. Please do not make me swab my quails!'

Should I have done a forensic investigation and swabbed my dead quails, I would most assuredly have found cat DNA, conclusively proving that my neighbour's ginger cat (and not some other random cat) had killed my quails. Anyway, I had seen the ginger cat slinking off out of my backyard, and that is how I knew it was the culprit. I never did swab the quails; I simply walked away, my mood low.

The following day I took a walk in the university garden to get some fresh air and contemplate my new, quail-less life. When things get too much, I like to walk and sit on the benches beneath the tall trees at my faculty, which has beautiful lawns. Sounds idyllic, doesn't it? Now remember, there is always a downside in life: when I stood up from the bench, waxy-white resin stained the posterior aspect of my trousers. The resin had been dripping silently from the over-hanging trees and as a result my trousers were ruined.

My quails. My trousers. What did they all have in common? Locard's Exchange Principle: every contact leaves a trace.

The world is complex and dynamic, with multiple systems at play. Everything is being interchanged on a macro- and microscopic scale. As you sit reading right now, you are being bombarded with stuff even though most of what is happening to you is imperceptible to your human sensory spectrum: light rays, dust particles with their Brownian motion, different frequencies of radiation, ultraviolet light and, of course, cell phone signals. (Brownian motion is the random motion of particles that are suspended in a fluid, a liquid or a gas, and results from their collision with the fast-moving atoms or molecules in the gas or liquid.) Chemicals are being transferred and interchanged everywhere; some chemicals will ultimately end up being swallowed – and you wonder how and why people get sick!

The law of interchange – Locard's Exchange Principle – is alive and well. It works on the cosmic scale and it works on the subatomic scale. It functions throughout our lives and in all arenas of our lives.

What is evidence? Physical evidence is any type of evidence with an objective existence – that is, anything with size, shape and dimension. Physical evidence can take any form: it may be as large as a house or as small as a fibre. It may be as fleeting as an odour or as obvious as the scene of an explosion. Evidence may have certain class characteristics: urine, spittle, saliva, faeces, vomit, tissue, hair etc.

Physical evidence can prove a crime has been committed. It can establish key elements of a crime; for example, it can place the suspect in contact with the victim or the crime scene. It can establish the identity of persons associated with the crime or it can help exonerate the innocent. Physical evidence can also corroborate a victim's testimony. A suspect confronted with physical evidence may make admissions or even confess. Physical evidence may be more reliable than eyewitnesses to crimes. Evidence is dynamic: it moves, and it transfers throughout our lives.

So, what is trace? Trace evidence deals with the minute transfers of materials that cannot be seen with the unaided eye. The handling and analysis of trace evidence require care and specialised techniques. How can this trace be linked to its origin or to another trace? These are some of the most important questions asked in this book.[1] When it comes to evidence (or trace evidence) collection, you only get one shot at the homicide crime scene, so you need to obtain as much information and document as much as possible. You seriously only get one bite at the cherry.

The process of trace evidence analysis is critical in catching murderers because the variety of material that may require analysis is almost without limit. At one time or another the renowned forensic scientist and pathologist Sir Sydney

Smith (1883–1969) obtained evidence from the examination of the following trace evidence: glass, sand, earth, paints, varnish, distemper, metal particles, oil, grease, lipstick and other cosmetics, polishes, woods, sawdust and vegetable matter such as algae and fungi.[2] In other words, Sir Sydney Smith used the aforementioned different types of trace evidence to catch murderers and solve crimes.

Frequently, several types of evidence require examination in the same case. Therefore, if someone is found dead, the ideal is to have detectives form a five-metre circle around the body, with each detective performing a finger-tip search with a magnifying glass as they all move closer and closer to the body. They may find footprints or cigarette butts or chewing gum lying about the body, for example. Forensic scientists are the ones who analyse, compare, evaluate and verify the evidence; they are the ones who actually solve the cases.

Evidence transfer, particularly trace evidence transfer, forms the basis of 'contact theory'.

3

Intensity, duration and nature
of the contact

One day in November 2021, I was called to a scene where a 41-year-old male construction worker had been found dead at approximately four o'clock in the afternoon. The man was found close to a housing development in the north of my jurisdiction. Scene examination showed a large amount of mud because of rain, and there were remnants of torn and tattered clothing.

Autopsy examination showed linear, longitudinally orientated scorch burns over the left side of the deceased's neck, the front of the chest, the left inguinal region and the inner aspect of the left thigh. The right eardrum was ruptured and the deceased's pubic hair was singed.

There was another unusual skin injury, which could not initially be explained, pertaining to an area measuring approximately 10 x 7 cm overlying the right side of the chest, where multiple small metallic elements from a metallic zipper could be seen on the skin, in relation to multiple small burn marks. Several of these metallic elements were melted and embedded into the skin. I had never seen anything like this before.

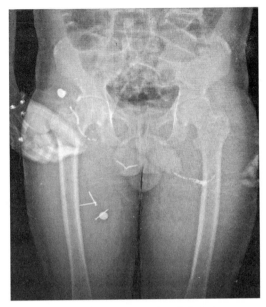

An X-ray showing three pieces of exploded zipper across
the construction worker's groin.

My examination of the man's internal organs didn't shed any further light on what could have been the cause of death. The torn and tattered clothing showed synthetic material melting at places. The front of the denims the man wore was covered with mud. There was a patch overlying the anterior aspect of the left thigh region, which showed tearing. Interestingly, the zipper on the front of the blue denims was damaged. I was intrigued by the unusual skin injury on the right side of the chest – the marks were suggestive of burns from elements from a damaged zipper. Ultimately, X-rays confirmed a damaged and 'exploded' zipper.

After scene examination and autopsy I had to conclude

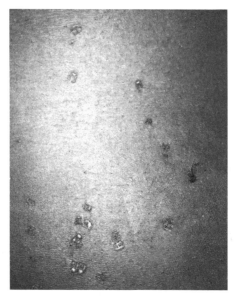

The teeth (elements) of the zipper had melted and embedded themselves into the victim's skin.

that the man had died from a direct lightning strike. How did I come to this conclusion? With my knowledge of Locard's Exchange Principle.

Even when an event takes place very quickly, we will be able to find evidence of its existence. In the case of lightning, it may strike too quickly for us to see what is really going on; however, lightning leaves clues. It leaves traces of itself. It tells one what has happened, what it is made from, its physics and its essence.

In a typical lightning strike investigation, we would begin by looking for damage to nearby trees – although one might not know what those trees looked like before the thunderstorm. While it will be difficult to date when exactly any damage to a tree occurred, the sudden onset of brown discoloration of leaves after a thunderstorm could be indicative of a lightning strike. When in doubt, we may submit leaves to a plant pathologist for review.

The ground may display a fern-like pattern that might be rather subtle. Soil may show fulgurite formation – that is, tube-like structures formed in sand or rock. Both the fern-like pattern and the fulgurite formation are caused by lightning. Often, a crater will be exposed in the earth, with rock and sand being flung far afield: craters of up to two metres in diameter have been reported. Other craters may be less obvious.

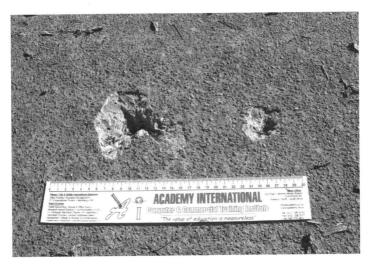

The effect of lightning striking a concrete pavement.

There is a misconception called the 'crispy-critter myth', because it is commonly thought that animals or birds struck by lightning will look like 'crispy critters', that is, charred pieces of carbonised remains – this is entirely false. The signs of lightning on a dead animal or bird may be very faint. Animal and bird lightning fatality cases may show scorched hair and/or feathers. The singeing of feathers may be subtle and only identifiable with an alternate light source or special filters for photomicrography.

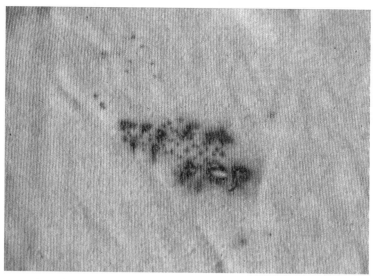

Holes densely arranged in groups are a typical effect of lightning strikes (comparable with lesions from shotgun pellets).

Findings on the clothing of lightning strike victims may show holes densely arranged in groups, comparable with lesions from shotgun pellets. Synthetic textiles may show uncharacteristic tears, as well as heat changes with local hardening and rolled-in margins with microscopically detectable melting effects (e.g. club-shaped fibre ends). Shoes often show tiny holes or tears in the sole or the adjacent upper aspects. Leather shoes may be violently torn, signifying the great forces at play during lightning strikes.

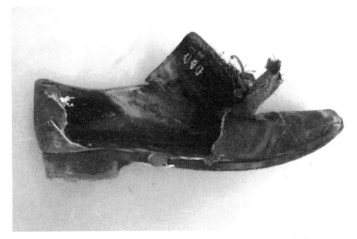

Lightning can even tear leather shoes apart, proof of the extreme forces at play.

Lightning may cause singed head hair, eyebrows, eyelashes, body hair and pubic hair. There may be clusters of punctate burns, blisters or charred burns on the skin. Extensive burns on the body surface are by no means a constant finding; often there may be no burns whatsoever.

The best-known finding on the skin in lightning strike victims is the so-called Lichtenberg figure, named after German physicist Georg Christoph Lichtenberg (1742–1799). Lichtenberg figures represent a vital reaction and are most commonly seen in light-skinned lightning strike survivors. They are reddish, fern-like (arboresque) skin patterns resulting from transient hyperaemia, which blanche or disappear

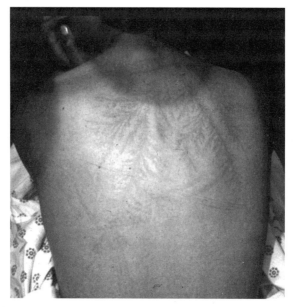

A Lichtenberg figure on the upper back of a person who was hit by lightning. Photo: Mary Ann Cooper, MD

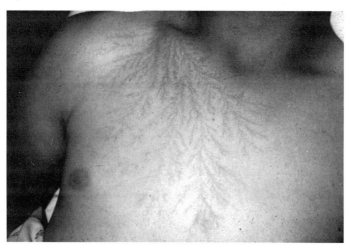

A Lichtenberg figure overlying a man's chest. Photo: Mary Ann Cooper, MD

after several hours. What this means is that victims basically look as if they have been slapped with a wet tree fern. Histologically, Lichtenberg figures consist of small, dilated vessels in the corium (the deeper, thicker layer of skin under the epidermis).

The ears must be checked for ruptured drums and for leaking blood. Eyes should also be checked: retinal detachment may be seen in acute cases, while cataract formation can be seen in lightning strike survivors. Cataracts typically develop a few weeks or even months after a lightning incident.

Small molten beads may be found on metallic elements of the victim's clothing, buckles and snap-fasteners, including watches and pieces of jewellery. This phenomenon is known as 'lightning metallization injury'.

Remember: every contact leaves a trace, which means we can deduce much about the nature of lightning by merely looking at what traces it leaves behind on the body. We notice that lightning is actually a multi-physics phenomenon. There may be light injury (which can affect the eyes), heat injury (which can cause burns), blast injury (which can rupture eardrums) or electrical injury (which can cause Lichtenberg figures).

So, back to the deceased construction worker: why did the victim's zipper explode during a lightning strike? Why did the metal elements melt, and how did they become embedded in the victim's skin? The melted zipper elements were lodged on the right side of his chest, and yet the zipper was located in the groin region.

The answer is that most necklaces and zippers are not solid, wire-like structures. Instead they are made up of

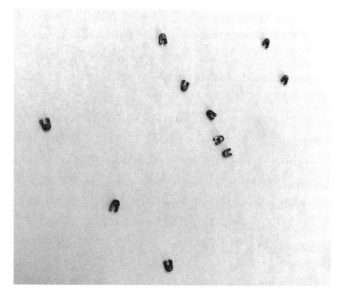

*A close-up photograph of the teeth (elements)
from the exploded zipper.*

several loosely connected links. Apart from melting the metal,
the intense lightning current may create micro-arcs across
these links, causing mechanical forces to rip the necklace
or zipper into several fragments. This phenomenon may be
likened to an explosion of the necklace or zipper: in other
words, the metallic zipper from the denims, which served as
a 'floating electrode', held on to the lightning's electric charge,
sparks jumped between the elements of the zipper, and then
the zipper heated up, exploded and melted into the skin of
the deceased.

The second part of Locard's Exchange Principle states that
the intensity, duration and nature of the materials in contact

32

determine the extent of the transfer. These are important considerations to keep in mind.

Intensity refers to the magnitude or degree of strength, force or energy. *Duration* refers to the length of time something continues. *The nature of the material* refers to what the material is composed of, or whether it is hard, soft, sharp or blunt.

For example, contact may be extreme and hard – or light and subtle. Needless to say, it is easier to detect extreme or hard contacts. The more experienced and advanced you become in forensics, the greater your chance of detecting subtle contacts.

When it comes to lightning injury, the intensity of the contact is very important. Did the victim sustain a direct strike, where all the lightning current travelled through the body? Or did the victim sustain a smaller dosage of lightning, where most of the lightning charge was dumped on the tree and he only sustained a smaller portion of the lightning dose?

The same applies to poisoning: someone may have significant exposure to a poison and die. Or the person could be exposed to small dosages of poison over time. Forensic pathologists always have to ask themselves: how intense was the dosage, over what period was the victim exposed to it, and what was the nature of the poison?

4

Via negativa

The first death scene I ever attended was at a flat in the central area of my jurisdiction, in July 2001. I accompanied my old professor to what would become known as the 'Adam and Eve Murder'.

'Odd that there are no flies,' I recall my professor remarking when we entered the scene.

According to news reports at the time, Santa Pretorius, a nurse, had been attacked in her flat by a young couple while she was asleep in front of the television. The couple were a 15-year-old girl and her 17-year-old boyfriend, who called themselves Adam and Eve Gardens. The nurse awoke when she was attacked and begged the two to let her live. They didn't relent and continued stabbing her, so persistently that when the knife broke, they even went to find a second. They ended up stabbing Santa 37 times. Still they were not done, and Adam decided to strangle her with a shoelace.

Their intent was then to dismember her lifeless body and flush it down the toilet, but they never carried out this macabre plan. In a letter Adam later wrote to Eve he said that he did not have the courage and had been 'too lazy'.

After the murder, they stole a firearm from a friend and used it to hijack a car. The two were arrested shortly after the hijacking.

The couple was sentenced to a total of 21 years in prison. However, the judge ordered that they should effectively serve 20 years for the gruesome murder. In passing sentence, the judge said that Santa Pretorius had died a cruel death and had been denied dignity while experiencing extreme pain and fear. The judge was of the opinion that the murder had not been planned in advance and recommended that the couple not be released on parole before serving 15 years of their sentences, and not before they had been rehabilitated. Adam was sent to the Baviaanspoort prison and Eve to the Kroonstad prison, which had facilities to accommodate youthful criminals.

According to their diaries, the couple had, especially in the last months before the murder, partaken in unrestricted sex, drugs and alcohol, and the two had shown no respect for any form of authority. Both apparently came from dysfunctional homes, and Adam had seemingly been let down by the school system, having been expelled from his first school for stealing money when he was only in grade two. The judge could not disregard the prominent role that drugs and alcohol had played in their crimes and how these substances had influenced their behaviours. [1]

What I will never forget from that particular death scene was my old professor's remark about the absence of flies. Flies typically find a body within about two to three hours after death. Admittedly July is wintertime in South Africa, so we certainly would have expected fewer flies than during the summer months. However, their total absence could only be explained by the fact that all the windows and doors of that small flat had been tightly sealed by the perpetrators. It was my first proper exposure to the concept of *via negativa*.

Via negativa is another important tool in our cognitive forensic toolkit. It means 'by way of negation'. This Latin phrase has its roots in Christian theology, where it was used to explain the nature of God by focusing on what God *is not*.[2] In his book *Antifragile: Things That Gain from Disorder*, Lebanese-American essayist and mathematical statistician Nassim Nicholas Taleb describes it as 'subtractive knowledge': when one knows what is wrong with more certainty than one knows anything else.[3]

Often what we do *not* find at autopsy is more important than what we do find. In other words, the absence of evidence can be of greater value than the presence of evidence. This means you should have an idea of what isn't there. For example: how would one know what may have been stolen from a deceased person in the case of a house robbery? You would assume that the average person has a mobile phone and a wallet or a purse, and hence, when these items are *not* present at a death scene, you can assume that they were stolen. This requires a special way of reasoning and looking at things and a mind-set of noticing what is not there. Always ask what is missing, what is absent, what is not being said, what is not being discussed and what is not being shown. Notice what is not there.

An unidentified skeleton with a gap between the front teeth offers an example of how *via negativa* may be used for identification purposes: in such an instance the skull must be compared with a photograph of the missing person thought to be the deceased. If the negative space – that is the shape of the gap between the teeth – is the same ante-mortem and post-mortem, this then allows one to connect the teeth from the ante-mortem records with the teeth of the skeleton. (Please note that if the photograph was from a 'selfie' on a mobile phone, then you might have to flip the image around.[4])

In *Missing & Murdered*, Professor Emeritus in the Department of Human Biology at the University of Cape Town Alan G Morris calls this technique the 'exclusion principle'. He tries to imagine himself being cross-examined by the most tenacious and aggressive prosecuting attorney in the business, and he asks himself, 'What do I absolutely know for sure, and what am I guessing at?'[5] Rather than saying that a skull belongs to a certain person or group, he will start by saying what the skull is not, and be careful about saying what the skull is. Morris also tends to use expressions like 'falls within the range of' and 'cannot be excluded from'. Importantly, he is not averse to saying, 'I don't know.'

Now, suppose a body is found lying in the African veld in midsummer and it is alleged that the person has been dead for five days. However, when you arrive at the scene of death, you notice zero insect activity: there are no flies and not even a single ant. As I have mentioned, flies typically find a dead body within an hour or so. This means the person cannot have been lying under the hot African sun, at that specific scene, for five days. It is more likely that the person has been recently killed and dumped at the scene, or perhaps killed and refrigerated, and then dumped at the scene. This is a classic case where absence of evidence – the absence of insect activity – could help solve the case.

Via negativa – looking for what is not there – is therefore a power weapon in your forensic cognitive toolkit.

A way in which we use *via negativa* in everyday life is by looking at what people do not elect to say and what they do not do. I am always surprised by people who order food and beverages but never say 'Please' or 'Thank you'. This happens more often than you might think. The absence of these important words tells me a lot about the particular person.

Sometimes, when I am undressing a body, I notice the absence of certain clothing. It fascinates me how many people do not wear underwear or socks. At times, this finding may be significant, for example in a drug-facilitated sexual assault, where the aggressor dresses the victim after the assault but omits the underwear. Sometimes what you don't find is more important than what you do find. I am also surprised by politicians and lobby groups who fail to condemn certain acts of violence, especially when they vociferously condemn others.

As a forensic pathologist, I see all types of violence. Some cases make the news, other cases do not. How can one case of violence be more deplorable than another? Unless, of course, you have some or other special agenda. To me, elder abuse is just as deplorable as child abuse, in that the victims in both cases are from vulnerable populations. However, there are far more campaigns against child abuse than there are campaigns against elder abuse.

5

Making decisions with minimal data

In December 2022, I had an unusual case concerning a young man of 19 with stab wounds from glass. At first, we didn't know what to make of the death scene.

The full story only came to light a while later, after interviews with the parents. Their son had locked himself in their bedroom and removed the gun from the safe in order to shoot himself. Apparently, the gun did not work, so he took off his belt and tried to hang himself. However, he found there was no point from which to suspend himself, so he broke the window and stabbed himself to death with a large piece of shattered window glass.

What we found at the scene certainly required some clarification and begged the question: was it an accident, suicide or murder? (Some countries even make provision for what they term 'misadventure'.) This is a crucial question that will automatically arise when any fatal wound is being examined. It demands that the investigation be approached with an open mind.

When assessing a wound, one has to employ a carefully planned procedure. Nothing must ever be taken for granted.

How does the investigator contend with substantiating cause of death? Or understand contributing factors?

One needs to gain a clearer picture of the sequence of events and try to understand what happened first. All decisions must be based on facts and the importance of 'hard evidence' must be emphasised.

The question is: how much data is required before you can solve a case? If you see something macroscopically – in other words, visible to the naked eye – can you diagnose it based on gross pathology alone or do you have to prove it with ancillary investigations, such as histology (the microscopic structure of tissues), immunohistochemistry (an auxiliary method used by pathologists to visualise the distribution and amount of certain molecules in the tissue using specific antigen-antibody reactions) or electron microscopy (a technique used to investigate the detailed structure of tissues, cells, organelles and macromolecular complexes)?

At what stage is one satisfied with the diagnosis? At what stage can you call it? In layman's language, if it looks like an elephant, can I diagnose an elephant? Or do I have to perform special investigations, such as DNA tests, to *prove* that it *actually is* an elephant? (There are in fact three species of elephant: the African savanna, or bush, elephant, the African forest elephant and the Asian elephant.) Is it not good enough for me to simply diagnose that it is an elephant?

To add to this, what does one do in a resource-depleted and resource-limited environment, where there is no immuno-histochemistry or electron microscopy? Can good medicine be practised with peanuts? This comes down to making

41

excellent decisions with minimal data. When you diagnose at autopsy, how much evidence do you need to say with absolute certainty: this is what it is?

Let's take herpes hepatitis or herpes simplex virus (HSV) hepatitis as an example to explain this point. Herpes hepatitis is a rare but frequently intense and severe disease of the liver. It most frequently affects immunocompromised patients. How far should I go to diagnose herpes hepatitis in a resource-limited or resource-depleted environment?

First described in adults in 1969, HSV hepatitis is an uncommon complication of herpes simplex infection that can lead to acute liver failure.[1] To the unaided eye, herpes hepatitis at autopsy may show necrosis of the liver. (Necrosis is the death of cells or tissue through disease or injury.) The deceased is usually a pregnant woman or an immuno-compromised patient. Approximately 58 per cent of cases can be diagnosed via histologic and immunohistochemical analysis of liver tissue.[2] Histology typically confirms the geographic (non-zonal) haemorrhagic necrosis. You could also use HSV immunostaining to diagnose the condition or employ diagnostic tools such as serology, polymerase chain reaction, computed tomography scan and liver biopsy. However, all of these tools cost money. Lots of money.[3]

There are many other pathologies which can look exactly like herpes hepatitis.[4] Therefore the question arises: how much money should you throw at such a case to diagnose it? Can you diagnose it with the naked eye alone or do you need fancy-schmancy equipment? Do you need microscopic examination, serology, polymerase chain reaction (PCR) and electron microscopy? At what stage will you be happy with your diagnosis? How much evidence do you really need to say that this is what it is?

What I am getting at is this: is it possible to solve a crime *cheaply* with minimal data?

Someone is found dead from a gunshot wound in the passageway of a house. There are no witnesses or history. (Again, there is minimal data.) In South Africa, it is not the function of the medical practitioner, but that of the courts (the magistrate or the judge), to establish whether a death was the result of murder, suicide or accident. This having been said, there are no witnesses or any discernible history to explain what has occurred. How would an expert know if this was a case of suicide, homicide or accident? How can Locard's Exchange Principle be used to help determine the manner of death here?

Start by drawing up a list of all the factors that could potentially make it most likely a suicide, an accident or a homicide.[5] Suicides, for example, typically happen in the bedroom or the bathroom, hardly ever the passageway. Suicidal gunshot wounds are typically tight-contact or loose-contact gunshot wounds. Suicide victims typically also aim for their head or heart. There are areas of predilection for suicidal gunshot wounds, such as the temple of the head, the inside of the mouth or below the chin. The site of election may vary with the length of the weapon used. In suicides, people rarely shoot themselves in the eye, the nose or the ear – it is almost as if they don't want to hurt themselves.

Furthermore, people rarely shoot themselves in inaccessible sites, such as the back. For most suicidal gunshot wounds, the angle of trajectory is typically upwards or horizontal: when someone shoots themselves, their arms typically sag, and the gunshot wound is aimed in an upward direction. Suicidal wounds are most often in accessible sites and within range of the deceased's arms (unless some device was used to reach and depress the trigger). The weapon is most often present at the scene, even though it may be a distance from the body if it has been catapulted away by the gun recoiling, or by movement of the body if death was not instantaneous. The deceased's DNA or fingerprints are usually present on the weapon, unless the deceased was wearing gloves.

Homicides, on the other hand, typically happen in any room of the house. The angle of trajectory for most homicidal gunshot wounds is typically horizontal or downwards: when someone is shot by another person, the arms of the shooter typically take aim, resulting in that angle. Multiple gunshot wounds suggest homicide – although an unusual case of suicide involving nine gunshot wounds to the anterior chest has been described in the literature. To date, I think this is the world record. This unusual case illustrates that individuals may continue to function for a short time with fatal wounds and underlines the importance of a complete investigation.[6]

Something else to be considered is the possibility of the

manner of death being staged. Staging may give the appearance of death having occurred as a result of an accident or suicide, whereas in fact it was murder. Staging is nothing more than a form of tampering, which I will discuss later in this chapter.[7]

One can perform a statistical process known as a forensiometric analysis, a new form of multivariate analysis introduced in 1999. It is possible to differentiate between firearm-related homicides and suicides using multivariate analysis.[8]

Probability theory (the branch of mathematics concerned with describing how likely an event is to occur) can also help solve crimes, based on Bayes' theorem, which updates the probability for a hypothesis as more evidence or information becomes available.[9] By applying probability theory – and therefore without the use of expensive equipment, in this instance! – you can get a clearer picture of whether a case is homicide, accident or suicide. This is a very powerful tool, especially when it comes to solving equivocal death scenarios, meaning a death that could be due to any number of reasons. Solving what once appeared to be an unsolvable case suddenly becomes easier.

So, even when you have limited data, you can still solve cases.

Accidental shootings have their own forensiometrics: Accidental shooting cases may be difficult to diagnose and typically fall in the grey area between cases that are classically homicidal and those that are classically suicidal. One such case was related to me by my old professor: apparently a teacher was casually showing another teacher his gun at a restaurant and, according to the first teacher, his gun 'accidentally went off'. At autopsy, there was a tight-contact gunshot wound to the chest. This was unlikely to be an accidental shooting case – because who shows a gun with it tightly pressed against the precordium of another's chest?

Russian roulette is another example. Russian roulette is a potentially lethal game of chance in which a player places a single round in a revolver, spins the cylinder, places the muzzle against the head or body of the opponent or themselves, and pulls the trigger. If the loaded chamber aligns with the barrel, the weapon will fire, killing or severely injuring the player. Some jurisdictions classify Russian roulette as 'accidental' or 'misadventure'. I would classify this lethal game as suicidal.

There are, of course, limits to Locard's Exchange Principle, and I want to mention these now in the context of evaluating data. Two questions should always be asked: Does absence of evidence equal evidence of absence? And, does presence of evidence equal evidence of presence?

In terms of the first question: just because something is not there, does that mean it was *never* there? Could it have been removed? Take rape, for example: the absence of certain injuries does not exclude rape. It can happen that no injuries are left on the external genitalia during a rape.

In terms of the second question: just because something is there, does that mean that it *really is* there, and always was, or might it have been placed there? Could something that has been found at the scene of a crime have been placed by someone with nefarious intentions? Using rape again as an example: the presence of injuries does not necessarily mean that a rape took place, because consensual sexual intercourse may sometimes leave injuries. Furthermore, the injuries could have been caused by the person themselves.

These questions require the mind-set of the forensic medical detective: rape is not only about finding semen, even though semen is good and strong evidence, given that it contains DNA. What happens if the rapist wore a condom? What happens if the rapist had a vasectomy? Semen without sperm still contains substances which may be identified, such as acid phosphatase and prostate-specific antigen. Prostate-specific antigen, found in semen, may also be transferred. Epithelial skin cells from the mucosal surfaces may be transferred. Even sexually transmitted diseases and lubricants on the outside of a condom may be transferred.[10] Therefore careful observation (noticing) is required of both what is present and what is not.

What, then, is tampering? To 'tamper' means to interfere with something in order to cause damage or make alterations. Evidence may be tampered with or contaminated, which is why the preservation of evidence is critical. Tampering is typically done surreptitiously.

It is a crime to wilfully destroy or hide evidence that is known to be relevant to a trial, police investigation, inquiry or other legal proceeding. So if someone removes evidence, or plants evidence, then subtle signs of the person who removed or planted the evidence must be sought out. This is where advanced forensics comes into play: one must seek evidence of the person who placed the false evidence or removed the actual evidence from the scene. Because even tampering leaves a trace!

Many murderers try to escape detection by making their crimes look like suicide or accident or natural death. One of the first cases in the literature was cited by my hero, Sir Sydney Smith, in his book *Mostly Murder*. He tells the story of how a gentleman called Sir Edmund Berry Godfrey 'was found impaled on his sword in 1678. At first sight it looked like suicide, as it was meant to. However, post-mortem examination showed that he had been strangled, and at the trial which ensued two surgeons testified that the sword-thrust was inflicted after death, and that his death was due to homicidal violence'. Three men were found guilty of Godfrey's murder and they were subsequently hanged.[11]

In one case I worked on, a young man had hanged himself. The parents were the first to come upon their son's body, and having found him in that state, they removed the noose, cleaned up the death scene, and placed him neatly in his own bed. The father phoned the police and reported the case as a sudden, unexplained death.

At autopsy, the signs of tampering on the body were so obvious to me: I could see the furrow mark on the neck, and I could even see an imprint of the point of suspension. I found the dried rivulet of saliva on the deceased's chest, indicating where the point of suspension of the noose would have been. I reported my suspicion to the detective, telling him that this had actually been a hanging case. I asked that he confront the family with this information and request that they reveal where they had hidden the noose. Upon questioning, the parents admitted that they had been embarrassed by their son's death – they said they thought it was cowardly of him to have taken his own life – so they tampered with the scene and placed him neatly in his own bed.

On another occasion, money that had been found in the clothing of a deceased individual was booked in as evidence. The next morning, the money was reported missing from the evidence collection bag, which had been in a safe. It was a matter of basic detective work to catch the culprit: who was on duty at the time? Who had access to the evidence collection bag? Who had access to the safe at that specific time? What did the CCTV footage show?

What the culprit had not realised was that I had recorded the serial numbers on the two-hundred-rand notes in my forensic report, so when one of the notes was found in his wallet, with an exactly corresponding serial number, it was like catching a fly with honey.

What happens when one comes across a death scene that seems overly complicated or appears to be unsolvable? There may be too little data or there may even be too much data. Furthermore, there may be a lot of media attention and perceived pressure to solve the case, and the people appointed to understand what has occurred may be left feeling overwhelmed.

When assessing a seemingly unsolvable case my advice is to work slowly. Gather all the facts. Focus on the inputs;

ignore the outputs. If one works diligently and thoroughly, the truth often spontaneously presents itself. And in cases where the pressure is immense or the case appears unsolvable, this is where experience and professionalism kick in.

I'd like to mention the concepts of wakefulness and watchfulness. One may not always be fully awake or fully watchful, nor might one notice everything or watch everything, especially when working long hours and when physical, mental and emotional exhaustion is taking its toll. This is when systemic methodology, processes and a good team will save you (particularly as a forensic pathologist) when you cannot save yourself.

There are some truly exceptional people in this field: they are profoundly present, seem to use all their senses, have keen insight and awareness, and are fully engaged in what they are doing – in fact, they almost seem to be cooking on more burners than average people. What happens when these exceptional people start running out of gas? How do they cook when they have no fuel or electricity, for that matter? Is it possible to still function optimally in such a scenario? Is it possible to practise forensic excellence when you are feeling fatigued from an increased workload?

If you look at the greatest forensic cases of all time, you'll see that hunches or intuition sometimes play a role: something likely strikes the investigator as being not quite right, and only later is science able to confirm the initial suspicions. Intuition and the good old hunch must not be discounted.

6

Looking for clues

In April 2021 I worked on a case where three people were found dead in a house and a fourth was alive, however, fighting for her life. A young woman was found dead, still seated, in a chair close to a door, while two men lay dead on the stairs leading to the bedroom.

There was no clear cause of death, making the scene examination incredibly difficult. So many things could have been responsible for their deaths because the average house contains a great many dangerous things. Initially, I suspected it might be a toxicological cause: some type of poison or gas. The cupboards in the house contained insecticides and pesticides and there were alcohol bottles at the scene, while the medicine cabinets were filled with a variety of weird and wonderful medicines: those to help with mental focus and concentration, and for anti-ageing and other forms of enhancement (designed to keep you 'forever young').

There was so much information to process, so many things to consider. It was only after the autopsy was completed that I would know that an overdose of an illicit drug – the date-rape drug gamma-hydroxybutyrate (GHB) – had killed them. GHB is a powerful, rapidly acting central nervous system depressant that was first synthesised in the 1920s and was used as an anaesthetic agent during the 1960s. It is produced naturally in the body, however, its physiological function is still somewhat unclear.

At the time of the deaths, GHB was not very common in South Africa and was very difficult to test for in forensic laboratories. However, I had read articles about GHB deaths in international journals and, based on these readings, decided to test for it.

GHB was sold as a performance-enhancing additive in bodybuilding formulas until it was banned by the United States Food and Drug Administration in 1990. Somehow, GHB entered the illicit market and began to be used for recreational purposes and in the dance club scene, specifically to enhance and prolong sexual sessions, as well as for drug-facilitated sexual assaults. GHB produces euphoric and hallucinogenic states and so it holds the potential for abuse, thereby representing a public health danger.

Some of GHB's street names are Chemsex, Cherry Meth, Fantasy, Georgia Home Boy, Great Hormones at Bedtime, Grievous Bodily Harm, Liquid E, Liquid Ecstasy, Liquid X, Organic Quaalude, Salty Water, Scoop, Sleep 500 and Vita G. It is produced in clandestine laboratories using inexpensive ingredients and from recipes taken off the internet.

It is clear, odourless, tasteless and usually taken orally in liquid form, so it will be undetectable when mixed in a drink. These are its effects according to dosage:

- 1 gram acts as a relaxant
- 2 grams causes strong relaxation
- 4 grams causes loss of motor and speech control

When mixed with alcohol, the depressant effects are enhanced. A coma-like sleep may therefore be induced, which is why it can be used in drug-facilitated sexual assault. The woman who survived and was in hospital had total amnesia.

GHB remains in the blood for four hours and is detectable in urine 72 hours after ingestion. It is typically hidden in eye-drop containers, so should a rapist who has used it be apprehended, the perpetrator will only have an eye-drop container on his person. 'Officer, all I have on me are these eye-drops for my red eyes!' they might say.

Date rape is also known as acquaintance rape, and both men and women can be targeted. Perpetrators look for a substance that is readily available and easy to administer, and that can produce loss of consciousness and retrograde amnesia. Four main date-rape drugs have typically been used: GHB, alcohol, benzodiazepines (e.g. Rohypnol) and ketamine.

Date rape often takes place against a background of some sort of illicit or recreational alcohol or drug use. There is typically no evidence of struggle and victims often report the crime late or may fail to report it at all. So, when dealing with such a victim, we need to know what symptoms to look for and how long the individual remained unconscious.

The classic date-rape drug is a sedative-hypnotic drug called flunitrazepam (better known by the brand name

Rohypnol) or roofies. It causes mild sedation and disorienta-
tion, but with increased dosage, a severe coma-like state may
result. Roofies produce dramatic muscle relaxation, slowing
of psychomotor responses, amnesia and disinhibition. They
may also be mixed with alcohol. Amnesia and blackout typically occur within 30 minutes to two hours after intake.
Hoffman-LaRoche, the company that produces Rohypnol,
reformulated it and the tablet now dissolves slowly in liquid
and releases a bright blue colour, so that a drink it has been
slipped into these days appears murky, and it is now detectable even in darker drinks. (It is important to keep in mind
that some date rapists may use old stock from before flunitrazepam was reformulated.)

Alcohol remains the most used and most abused substance in the world. Alcohol too has been utilised in date
rape, while alcohol poisoning and intoxication are very common. Even seemingly innocuous low-alcohol drinks can be
surreptitiously spiked with additional alcohol.

With alcohol at a blood alcohol concentration of 300–
350 mg/100 ml, you can expect stupor, coma and the danger of aspirating vomit. At blood alcohol levels above
350 mg/100 ml, there is a significant danger of death from
respiratory centre paralysis.

Alcohol is easily miscible with water. Hence people with
higher fat stores will produce higher blood-alcohol levels than
persons of the same weight who are lean. It is because of this
fact that women, due to their panniculus adiposus or higher
fat storage, may develop blood alcohol concentrations that
are 25 per cent higher than men of the same weight after
similar drinks.

Ketamine is a veterinary anaesthetic with amnesic actions lasting several hours that has been used by rapists to incapacitate their victims. Ketamine powder is sometimes snorted like cocaine and it may be applied to material that is smoked or consumed in a drink.

Considering date-rape drugs from the perspective of a Locard's Exchange Principle, whenever we as forensic experts have a possible victim of drug-facilitated sexual assault, we must notify the laboratory to urgently request a drug screen so as to identify which of the above substances may have been administered. However, interpretation is tough. We need to be able to answer the following questions: Was a drug or poison present or absent? What sort of action could the substance have exerted on the donor of the sample? Was the drug present in sufficient quantity to affect the behaviour or well-being of the donor of the sample? Could the substance have been influencing the donor at the time of the alleged incident?[1] In other words, we have to consider intensity, duration and nature of contact.

Illegal drugs are dangerous and constitute a lucrative business that harms society (both the victims and the perpetrators of drug-related crime) in multiple ways. When examining bodies, I always keep drugs in mind, because a victim of violence or crime may have been under the influence of a drug when they were harmed, injured or killed.

I had the following case brought to me. A 53-year-old male foreign national died suddenly and unexpectedly in a church. According to the man's brother, he was a very religious man,

55

attending church every day, sometimes three times per day. The CCTV footage showed the man dropping dead in the antechamber of the church.

Upon autopsy, I found a physically healthy-looking adult male with no fatal external injuries to the body. There were no scars, no tattoos, no needle puncture marks, nothing extraordinary. All his organs looked perfectly healthy, until I opened his stomach: it was filled with approximately 300 ml of white semi-digested, farinaceous (starch-like) food residue. I found three things within the stomach contents: a 20 cm length of sticky tape, a piece of twine and a small plastic bag. I made the diagnosis: what had killed the man was a ruptured 'drug bullet'.[2] I was dealing with a body-packer or stuffer, more commonly known as a drug mule.

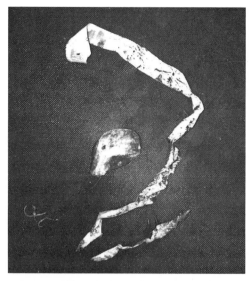

The ruptured drug package that was discovered in the stomach of a drug mule. It consisted of piece of Sellotape, twine and plastic wrapping.

People who have undertaken these jobs have been known to conceal drugs in their vaginas, rectums, mouths, ears, noses – even under their foreskins. As much as a kilogram of cocaine in a single load has been described in the literature. Loperamide, sold under the brand name Imodium, is generally used to decrease their gut motility. At journey's end, the mule takes laxatives for the drugs to pass. These drug packages are typically 25 mm x 15 mm in size. Typically condoms, balloons or the distal ends of rubber glove fingers are used.

Sometimes the drug cartel marks the courier's buttocks with the pointed end of a knife, creating a human invoice pad: ten knife-point wounds are equivalent to ten swallowed drug bullets. This human invoice-pad technique prevents the mules from cutting out the drug dealer or dealing on the side. These drug packages or drug bullets may leak, resulting in an overdose or death, as in the case of the foreign national patient. (Another possibility is that the person I examined swallowed the drugs immediately before a perceived arrest, and the drugs were not well wrapped.)

Here is another tragic scenario. A recently arrived foreign national is found dead in a transients' hotel (near an airport, train station or harbour). The death scene shows laxatives nearby. Interestingly, the radiodensity of heroin and cocaine is very close to that of stool on X-ray examination. This is why clinicians sometimes use CT scanning or barium contrast studies to demonstrate the presence of these drugs.

Cocaine causes terminal hyperthermia (high temperatures), which is why, at the scene of death, the body may typically

57

be covered with wet towels or ice may be strewn about. Sometimes the body is found under an air-conditioner or fan. Heroin causes foaming around the mouth and nostrils.

There are reported cases of the body having been cut open by the cartels to retrieve the drugs at the death scene. The couriers are often entirely expendable to their traffickers. These drug cartels are usually quite sophisticated and some even own their own cell phone networks and satellite phone systems.

There are always newer and more cunning techniques of transporting drugs through customs. Officials would not be surprised to find a woman with breast implants containing pure cocaine or heroin instead of silicone. Other craftier methods include packing the drugs subcutaneously inside surgical wounds and suturing the wounds closed. There have even been cases of pets being used to transport drugs, surgically sutured under the skin of a dog or cat: a whole new, wicked way to exploit pets.

The medical management of surviving drug mule suspects, who have been caught by the police, is controversial. Some doctors surgically remove the packages, while other doctors wait for them to pass.

Drugs are also commonly used in cases of suicides, and increasingly those of very high-profile individuals. One of the most famous drug-related deaths was, of course, that of Marilyn Monroe. The forensic pathologist who performed Monroe's autopsy was Thomas Tsunetomi Noguchi, who served as Chief Medical Examiner-Coroner for the County of Los Angeles from 1967 to 1982. Known as the 'coroner to the stars', Noguchi performed autopsies on Robert F Kennedy, Sharon Tate, William Holden, Natalie Wood, John Belushi and Gia Scala.

I was deeply honoured to meet Noguchi, one of my forensic heroes, in Minneapolis in September 2016 when I attended one of the premier forensic pathology conferences in the world, that of the USA's National Association of Medical

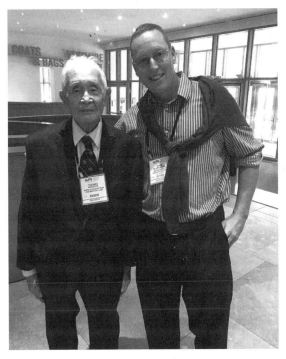

The author with renowned forensic pathologist and 'coroner to the stars', Thomas Tsunetomi Noguchi , who served as the Chief Medical Examiner-Coroner for Los Angeles County.

Examiners. I was the only forensic pathologist representative from South Africa (or Africa, for that matter) at that particular conference.

On the autopsy of Marilyn Monroe, Noguchi said the following about this high-profile death: 'In 1962, an actress named Marilyn Monroe, who was 36 years old at the time and a superstar in Hollywood, was found dead while nude in her bedroom. My chief, Theodore J Curphey, assigned the case to me. The autopsy revealed the cause of death to be an overdose of barbiturates (sleeping pills). In LA County, this was the first case where we used psychological autopsy to investigate a death. After declaring it a suicide by overdose of barbiturates, we were challenged by the news media. Even now, after 50 years, I still receive inquiries from journalists who are interested in writing books.'[3]

Interestingly, *Quincy, M.E.*, also called *Quincy*, the American mystery medical drama television series from Universal Studios that aired on NBC from 1976 to 1983, was probably based on the career of Dr Thomas Noguchi. Jack Klugman starred in the title role as a Los Angeles County medical examiner who routinely engaged in police investigations.

On a personal note, attending the conference was a huge responsibility in my eyes and I presented a poster which was relatively well received. There were several highlights during this conference: the lectures were all of a very high standard, I learned so much, I met my heroes whose books I had studied, and I was even invited to attend the 90th birthday celebrations of Thomas Noguchi. Being a forensic pathologist certainly has its highlights.

CASE STUDY 1

A 45-year-old male was taken to an emergency room after he had drunk methylated spirits. He arrived at the hospital in an encephalopathic (brain-damaged) state, and his condition quickly deteriorated.

He was declared brain dead the following day. An autopsy examination demonstrated bilateral putaminal haemorrhages – bleeding on the outer part of the lentiform nucleus of the brain. It was deemed an unnatural death and a medico-legal autopsy was arranged to be performed the following day, in accordance with the national regulations.

The autopsy showed no fatal external injuries to the body. The brain was pale and weighed 1 386 grams. Serial sections of the brain showed bilateral globus pallidus haemorrhages. These acute haemorrhages were also confirmed on histology.

Methylated spirits, a denatured alcohol, is also known as wood alcohol and is typically used as a cleaning agent for household purposes. It may be made unpalatable by mixing it with other, often toxic, chemicals to prevent recreational abuse. Symptoms and survival time are determined by the amount ingested.

The combination of visual damage and bilateral putaminal necrosis is pathognomonic of methanol intoxication; this means that these findings are distinctive or characteristic and enable a diagnosis to be made. Methanol causes destruction of myelin in the optic nerve, which may lead to permanent visual problems. The 45-year-old male did not report any visual disturbances.

Once methanol is consumed and has reached the organs, it is converted through a series of steps into formic acid. Eventually formic acid will be formed into carbon dioxide and water. This last reaction is rather slow, which leads to an accumulation of formic acid, which is toxic to humans.

There are multiple hypotheses as to why specifically the putamen (the outer part of the lentiform nucleus of the brain) is affected by methanol poisoning while other structures of the brain stay intact. One hypothesis suggests that putaminal neurons show a higher sensitivity to acidic environments and therefore are more affected by formic acid than other structures of grey matter.

Almost everything leaves traces of itself. In this instance, methylated spirits left traces of itself on the globus pallidus. A formal meeting with the deceased's sister, one day after death, presented us with the history that he had been drinking methylated spirits. This case happened during Covid-19 lockdown, when there were alcohol restrictions.

CASE STUDY 2

Pathognomonically speaking, Temik poisoning is a South African way to die. Also known as Two-Step (step one, you swallow it; step two, you die) or Haliparemi, it is a pesticide that contains the active ingredient aldicarb. It is a type of organophosphate poison (organophosphates are used as insecticides and nerve agents) and it is a common way for burglars to poison dogs in South Africa. Symptoms of Temik poisoning include increased saliva and tear production, diarrhoea, vomiting, small pupils, sweating, muscle tremors and confusion.

Sadly, we see many cases of temic poisoning on our autopsy tables. (As an aside, I wonder if my international colleagues would be able to diagnose this macroscopically.) The victims are typically well-dressed men in their mid-twenties or mid-thirties who are 'found dead', with no further history. There would be no suicide notes or any-

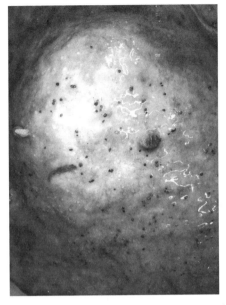

The multiple small pepper-like granules within the stomach contents are Temik (aldicarb), commonly known as 'Two-Step'.

thing else at the death scene to alert the detectives, to whom the cause of death will likely appear to be quite a mystery.

At autopsy, upon external examination, the first thing I notice is faecal staining of the buttocks. There are typically no other external injuries on the person. When I open the stomach, I am hit by the strong chemical odour. Then, admixed within the stomach contents, I notice multiple, small, poppy-seed-like granules. Temik is widely used as a pesticide on crops such as cotton, potatoes and peanuts. As aldicarb is a member of the carbamate pesticides, these small grey-black granules are highly toxic.

Even though it looks like suicide, I am always struck by the absence of any suicide note. I have literally never ever seen a Temik case with a suicide note and neither have any of my colleagues. This tells me – *via negativa*! – that something else is probably at play here. Despite my questioning many people over many years, no one has ever been able to give me a satisfactory answer. Was the victim who ingested the Temik perhaps misinformed about the substance itself? Or was the Temik sold to the victim under false pretences? Did the person taking the Temic maybe think it was a special medicine to make him stronger, or perhaps 'cleanse' him, or perhaps enhance him in some way or other?

7

Almost everything leaves a trace

Some gases pose a real danger to members of the public, and also to forensic pathologists, a number of whom have been injured by gases.

Once a colleague of mine was tasked to perform a repeat autopsy on a body from a private undertaking company. Three mortuary technicians winched the lid off the wooden coffin, which had been tightly sealed with metal screws. As they opened the coffin, all three were overcome by toxic gas, and soon thereafter were rushed to hospital. They developed pulmonary oedema from chemical injury to their lungs. Two were discharged within the week, the third spent three weeks in hospital.

What was the chemical gas which had so injured my colleagues?

The private undertaker had learned that a cup of granulated chlorine placed in a mortuary fridge would dispel unpleasant odours. (It is magical stuff and works better than most sprays or fragrances.) The undertaker adopted this method and developed the secret practice of sprinkling granulated chlorine into coffins around deceased individuals. In

retrospect, once can hardly blame the person for his inge-
nuity; his motto, after all, was to deliver 'a clean and serious
service'.

What the undertaker did not take into consideration was
that when a body decomposes, purge fluids are released,
which tend to react with the chlorine granules, creating chlorine gas. Chlorine gas is pale green, irritant and toxic: it's
dangerous and even deadly.

One of the most toxic gases is formaldehyde, which is used
to preserve tissues. Long-term inhalation of formaldehyde
has been associated with an increased risk for all cancers of
the lung and nasal passages.[1]

Forensic pathologists and mortuary technicians are sometimes also exposed to cyanide when performing autopsies
on persons who have ingested this substance.[2] Although
cyanide can volatilise from autopsy tissues, the major risk to
autopsy personnel occurs when the stomach is opened. In
the acidic environment, cyanide salts are converted to highly
volatile hydrocyanide gas.

Exposure to gastric contents and clothing contaminated
with organophosphate poisoning can be dangerous too.[3]
Poisoning can be very surreptitious. There have even been
cases of people being poisoned from chair covers which had
been contaminated by poison during transport.[4]

In May 2011, I had to deal with a complex case involving an
unknown poison that had killed an electrical apprentice who
had been contracted to perform electrical maintenance work
of a general nature at the premises of a bus transport company in Mbombela.

The facility included two wash bays where the buses were cleaned by an outside cleaning contractor. The buses were cleaned using water, cleaning detergents and chemicals. Fluids drained from the wash bays through underground pipes, via two sand traps where the heavier residue was removed and the residual fluid – comprising a mixture of water, detergents and chemicals, including some oil residue – collected in an underground pit.

There was a second, shallower pit situated about two metres away, where a hydraulic pump was placed and used to pump the fluids from the pit into a separator, so water and oils were separated and drained off. At some point, the hydraulic pump became dysfunctional. Electrical contractors attended the premises a few days prior to the incident, at which time they installed a new electrical submersible pump. Thereafter it was noted that there was a fluid leak from a pipe leading to the pump, and an electrician was called to tighten a clamp on this leaking pump.

Mr J, the apprentice, was accompanied by a colleague, Mr R, to tighten the clamp on the leaking pipe. After arriving at the premises, Mr J removed his clothing and, wearing only a pair of shorts and gumboots, climbed down to the bottom of the five-metre deep pit. Mr J wore no safety clothing and had no breathing apparatus. His colleague remained outside the pit at the open manhole in order to pass tools down to him.

Apparently, Mr J developed some difficulty and bent over with his hands on his knees. He then either fell back or moved backwards into a sitting position in the fluid that was at the bottom of the pit. A short while later, he fell back-wards and lay on his back in the fluid. Mr R then called for assistance. Several employees arrived and entered the pit in order to remove Mr J (who was still alive at the time). Apparently, Mr J was lying on his back with the fluid level approximately at his chin and around his face.

One of the rescuers also developed breathing difficulties, and he too was pulled out of the pit and given some medical treatment but recovered immediately without any injury or ill-effects. An advanced life-support paramedic concluded that both Mr J and the rescuer had suffered the same condi-tion. A member from the fire and rescue service with 18 years' experience extracted the body of Mr J while wearing a breath-ing apparatus.

After Mr J was removed from the pit, he was put on a res-pirator to assist his breathing and was taken to hospital, where he was placed on a ventilator and life support. At the hospital, the medical practitioner, in her first report, wrote, 'patient collapsed due to toxic damps'. The internal medicine physician reported that Mr J was clinically brain-dead upon arrival. In his opinion, Mr J probably inhaled a volatile gas. Precisely what the gas was, however, remained unascer-tained at the time. Mr J's condition deteriorated and two days later, the life support was switched off.

Witnesses speculated that there had been possible gas-eous exposure. Could it have been carbon monoxide, hydro-gen sulphide or even hydrochloric acid? All were considered and the fire department was asked to take gas readings in the pit. The readings for carbon monoxide, chlorine and hydrogen sulphide were low and the gases deemed not to be present.

I was consulted as an expert forensic pathologist and was shown the CCTV footage, which recorded the following sequence of events (showing minutes and seconds elapsed from the start of the recording):

09:32 – Car arrives.

11:43 – Mr J undresses and appears to move and function relatively well. Mr J enters the pit.

13:03 – Colleague runs to get help.

14:05 – Six helpers initially arrive at the pit.

16:44 – A ladder is brought to the scene.

18:55 – More than twenty onlookers surround the scene.

21:34 – Another car arrives.

23:00 – The first car leaves the scene.

25:16 – Paramedics arrive.

25:45 – Two further paramedic vehicles arrive.

27:00 – Another two paramedic vehicles arrive.

35:47 – The fire department vehicle arrives.

41:18 – A further ladder is placed into the pit.

47:00 – Mr J is removed from the pit and is resuscitated.

59:00 – Mr J is placed in the ambulance and the vehicle departs.

A sample of the water in the oil separator was sent for analysis. The following substances could be identified in the sample: aluminum, boron, calcium, potassium, manganese, nickel, phosphorous and zinc. The laboratory report also noted the presence of hydrogen sulphide gas in the sample (strong reaction). Hydrochloric acid liquid, mist or gas could also have been present.

Laboratories have developed tests that target sulphide and thiosulphate to detect hydrogen sulphide exposures. Hydrogen sulphide causes the atmospheric corrosion of copper. If a person is carrying copper-containing items (coins, keys, etc.) at the time of exposure and those items have changed colour, it is one possible indication that the person has been exposed to hydrogen sulphide.[5]

I performed the clinico-pathological correlation (CPC, an objective summary and correlation of clinical findings compared with the results obtained at autopsy) on this matter, and I suggested carbon dioxide to be the culprit agent for the following reason: carbon dioxide uses up space in the air instead of oxygen, creating an environment for asphyxiation. Findings in the history, CCTV footage and autopsy report were all in keeping with the possibility of carbon dioxide intoxication or poisoning.

Although much less abundant than nitrogen and oxygen in Earth's atmosphere, carbon dioxide is an important constituent of our planet's air. A molecule of carbon dioxide is made up of one carbon atom and two oxygen atoms. While carbon dioxide poisoning is rare, a high concentration in a confined space can be toxic. Carbon dioxide is colourless and, at low concentrations, odourless. At higher concentrations it may have a sharp, acidic odour.

Carbon dioxide poisoning is extremely difficult to prove or disprove at autopsy. It requires an insight into the situation, and often carbon dioxide poisoning occurs in areas and facilities far away from first-world forensic investigators and state-of-the-art medico-legal institutions. Even in the best medico-legal facilities around the world, the diagnosis of acute carbon dioxide poisoning would prove a challenge.

The autopsy findings in acute carbon dioxide poisoning are extremely non-specific. Signs suggestive of asphyxia or suffocation may be present: cyanosis, dark and fluid blood, congestion, oedema (build-up of fluid leading to swelling) and petechial haemorrhages (pinpoint collections of blood varying in size). If the victim survives for a few days and then dies from complications, the autopsy findings would be even more obscure, mainly because systemic complications, such as multiple organ failure, would most certainly be present.

Deaths from vitiated (spoiled, corrupted or impaired-quality) atmosphere are often due to carbon dioxide. Large quantities of carbon dioxide induce an oxygen deficiency. Carbon dioxide is not itself poisonous, however, it is irrespirable (incapable of being breathed). It may accumulate in fires, and in wells and shafts in limestone. In former years, vagrants sleeping for warmth near limekilns were sometimes suffocated by this heavy gas creeping over them.[6] The gases that accumulate, or that are fed into silos, wine cellars, breweries and tanks, can significantly reduce the oxygen content of the air, leading to rapid asphyxiation.

A carbon dioxide concentration of eight per cent by volume and above is potentially lethal.[7]

There are many instances where this happens in the natural world and when carbon dioxide from volcanoes creeps down towards low-lying areas. In relatively high concentrations, and without the dispersing effects of wind, it tends to collect in pocketed locations, because carbon dioxide is heavier than air.

A *mazuku* (the Swahili word for 'evil wind') is a pocket of carbon dioxide-rich air that can be lethal to any human or animal life. *Mazuku* winds are created when carbon dioxide accumulates in pockets low to the ground. A *mazuku* can be related to volcanic activity or to limnic eruptions, leading to several animals being affected: a zebra wanders into such a *mazuku* and dies due to asphyxiation, upon which a vulture, seeing the carcass, descends upon it and also dies. This situation has been witnessed in many species in the Virunga National Park in the Albertine Rift Valley in the eastern part of the Democratic Republic of the Congo.

On 21 August 1986, a limnic eruption at Lake Nyos in north-western Cameroon killed 1 746 people and 3 500 head of livestock. It became known as the Lake Nyos disaster.

Apparently, the eruption triggered the sudden release of about 100 000 to 300 000 tons of carbon dioxide. The gas cloud initially rose at nearly 100 kilometres per hour and then, being heavier than air, descended onto nearby villages, displacing all the air and suffocating people and livestock within 25 kilometres of the lake. The victims died of carbon dioxide asphyxiation.

A degassing system has subsequently been installed at the lake, with the aim of reducing the concentration of carbon dioxide in the waters and therefore the risk of further eruptions.[8]

Carbon dioxide is also the cause of deaths in a modern agricultural setting: the grain silo. Individuals can suffocate to death in a grain bin. Silo-filler's disease is the name given to the injury resulting from exposure to silo gas.

Many tons of grain are stored in gas-tight towers; the seed produces carbon dioxide that settles to the bottom of the tower. When a blockage occurs in the gravity discharge, farm workers may enter the tower to clear the obstruction. Although safety precautions demand venting before the men enter, some workers still suffer sudden death when encountering an atmosphere rich in carbon dioxide.[9]

To some adults, breweries may represent a modern-day Disneyland. However, even breweries can be deadly. Carbon dioxide is a necessary by-product in the brewing process, which means it can be a potential death trap for those working in the brewing industry. Duties such as cleaning fermentation tanks, maintaining yeast disposal and working in walk-in coolers are normal, daily, brewery activities – yet all are potentially hazardous spaces for brewery employees.

Dry ice is solid, frozen carbon dioxide, and, sadly, it has been used by individuals to commit suicide. For example, a person could lock themselves in the bathroom and seal the door. There may even be an advance directive on the outside of the bathroom door: 'Be careful when entering. Gas!' If they place a chunk of dry ice on the floor and lie down next to it, they will soon die. When first responders arrive at the scene, the chunk of dry ice may already have sublimated or evaporated. The person is simply found dead on the floor with no explanation.

Autopsy examination will prove non-specific and histology will also not help with your diagnosis. Neither will toxicology give you an adequate answer. If you are unaware of this phenomenon, you will most likely not be able to diagnose it. Not reading the academic literature and not knowing of such a phenomenon will cause many to miss the diagnosis. [10]

CASE STUDY 1

The damp steel walls of rusty old ships use up the oxygen, forming ferric oxides. Rust is a form of iron oxide, and it forms slowly when iron is exposed to air. This hazard exists in ships' tanks or other industrial metal chambers, in which oxygen is replaced by nitrogen.

This happens because the damp steel walls become rusty and use up much of the contained oxygen in forming ferric oxides.

In deaths associated with the replacement of oxygen by an inert gas, death is typically rapid. Bernard Knight, a legend in forensic pathology, mentions two deaths in which seafarers entered closed ships' tanks and virtually fell dead off the entry ladder. The presumed mechanism of death, which was far too quick to be hypoxic (low levels of oxygen), was considered to be due to some overstimulation of the chemoreceptor system (chemoreceptors are special nerve cells that detect changes in the chemical composition of the blood and send information to the brain to regulate cardiovascular and respiratory functions) leading to a parasympathetic vasovagal cardiac arrest (which is the stimulation of the parasympathetic system, causing slowing of the heart rate with a corresponding fall in the pulse rate). [11]

Breathing a gas mixture with no oxygen at all, such as pure nitrogen in the case of rusted old ships, can lead to loss of consciousness without the victim ever experiencing air hunger.

———————

Another gas that is difficult to detect is barium. 'Before you bury 'em, do a barium!' is a catchy, darkly humorous phrase coined by forensic pathologist Kathryn Pinneri, who is the director of Montgomery County Forensic Services in the United States. You can only diagnose what you test for in forensic medicine and pathology. If you don't think about it, you won't test for it, and consequently, you will not be able to diagnose it, hence the saying.

Fatalities can occur with the ingestion of soluble barium compounds. There are case reports of serious illness and fatalities in people intentionally or unintentionally exposed to barium carbonate or chloride. Ingestion of certain forms of barium in toxic amounts can lead to gastrointestinal signs and symptoms. Routine post-mortem toxicology panels may not always have barium as a commonly detected substance. This is why forensic pathologists must specifically request certain tests if they suspect certain poisons.

8

Specific contacts leave specific traces

A 45-year-old investment consultant whom I shall call Mr H had completed 19 Comrades Marathons, three Dusi Canoe Marathons, two Fish River hikes and two Drakensberg Challenge Canoe Marathons. The father of two was described as fit and healthy. He and three of his friends were part of a cycling group.

One Sunday morning, they departed from a shopping centre at approximately 07:20, heading towards a popular mountain bike area in the Cradle of Humankind. The group had been cycling for about ninety minutes before they turned back, taking a dirt road on their return. The path was well worn, however, before long the lead cyclist noticed that thick black power cables directly in their path were hanging extremely low. He braked sharply, shouting to the rest of his group to do the same.

Two more cyclists passed clear under the power line, but Mr H did not manage to react in time. He screamed, and when the three other cyclists turned round, they realised that their friend was locked into the cable. He was still on his bicycle and was entangled and being electrocuted.

The riders tried to pull Mr H free from the cable, yet despite wearing thick cycling gloves, felt the force of the electric shock as they tried to wrestle his body free. So strong was the surge of electricity, it knocked one of the cyclists off his feet. By this time, Mr H's clothing had started burning down one side. The three friends managed to manoeuvre his bicycle by holding on to the rubber tires and handlebar grips until he fell to the ground and was finally freed of his bicycle and the cable electrocuting him.

They extinguished the flames by rolling him over. Mr H was staring straight ahead, his jaw was clenched and he appeared not to be breathing. The men tried to clear his airway and attempted cardiopulmonary resuscitation. After about two minutes, Mr H began to breathe spontaneously, although laboriously.

With him breathing again, the cyclists understood the urgency of getting him to a hospital as soon as possible: they tried to call an ambulance, but unsuccessfully. They then attempted to carry him to the nearest road, yet only covered fifty metres or so, given that one of the men was still weak and shaky from being shocked. They managed to reach an abandoned house, and eventually one of them flagged down a car that could take Mr H to hospital. They arrived at the hospital at approximately 10:00.

Emergency help in the wild is about doing what you can, with what you have, where you are. There really was nothing else his friends could have done in that situation.

Mr H's admission records stated: 'Cycling this morning and cycled into a live electrical cable. Sustained burns. Brought in by ambulance. Male patient brought by friend per private transport with history of electrocution while cycling, trapped under hanging loose cables. Burns to right ear, right arm (from elbow to scapula), right thigh and bilateral inner aspects of thighs.'

Mr H sustained severe full-thickness electrical burns to the right forehead, neck, face, right ear, chest, arms and both thighs. As a result of the injuries, he experienced moderate to severe pain, suffering and discomfort for several weeks. He underwent medical treatment for some weeks, including multiple surgical debridement (removal of damaged tissue or foreign objects from a wound) and wound dressings. Cleaning and dressing of wounds occurred for approximately a further forty days after the surgeries.

Mr H survived the electrocution incident; however, he experienced disability and severe facial and bodily scarring in the areas where he had sustained the burns. According to reports, he experienced loss of earnings, loss of earning capacity and severe psychological shock and trauma.

People can get electrocuted in many different circumstances. I am going to discuss a typical forensic examination of an electrocution case to illustrate how a medical detective thinks about these kinds of cases.

In July 2010, an 11-year-old child was sitting in front of a PlayStation unit at a popular restaurant when he suddenly started convulsing. As the consulting forensic pathologist, I was given CCTV footage of the incident that showed the following:

14:45:58 – The child stands up from the chair.

14:46:14 – The child suddenly rotates anti-clockwise (twice).

14:46:19 – The child sustains blunt force trauma to the right parietal aspect of the head against the opposite aisle's television monitor.

14:46:21 – The child falls to the floor.

14:46:28 – The first responder comes to assist. The second responder arrives moments later.

14:46:45 – The child is seen to suffer tonic-clonic convulsions where the arms and legs begin to jerk rapidly and rhythmically, bending and relaxing at the elbows, hips and knees.

14:48:43 – The third responder comes to assist.

14:49:36 – A staff member is seen to be fanning the child.

14:54:21 – Everyone departs the scene.

The child survived and was taken to the nearest emergency room. He was drowsy and an examination showed that he was experiencing headaches and mild dizziness. There was no incontinence. At a physical examination the following morning, the child was alert and cooperative and had no further problems. Bite marks were present on the tongue and he had a bruise on the forehead.

A tiny one-millimetre white mark was present on the tip of the left index finger. However, I was not convinced that the lesion was electrothermal in origin. The child complained of a headache and backache, yet was neurologically intact.

I was consulted in my capacity as a 'skilled medical man

with a background in science' and asked by the lawyers whether this was a case of electrocution or epilepsy. If it was electrocution, there was a huge claim to be made against the popular restaurant. An epileptic-type seizure may sometimes be confused with an electrocution event.

An electroencephalogram (EEG) report indicated no obvious epilepsy. However, a mild abnormality was picked up which could possibly have predisposed the child to develop epilepsy. He was allegedly taking Ritalin for concentration problems. The same EEG changes had been present two years prior to the incident and were not new. (The subtleties and nuances of seizures and epileptic events are for the neurologist, so I won't delve into them.)

The fact that the body of the child convulsed on the floor for a period of seconds as people touched the child was critical to this matter, and could be witnessed on the CCTV footage. There were no reports or statements in the reports of anyone else feeling an electric shock while in physical contact with the body. (Extrication is usually extremely dangerous in an electrothermal event, as patients still in contact with a source of voltage usually transmit an electric current to would-be rescuers.) Scene examination of the gaming area showed electrical equipment (stripped, twisted connections, socket outlets, exposed wiring, etc).

This was a classic case of the fallacy expressed in Latin as *Post hoc, ergo propter hoc*, which means 'After this, therefore because of this,' or, in other words, since event Y followed event X, event Y must have been caused by event X. The logical fallacy of this lies in drawing certain conclusions solely on the basis of the order of events without considering other factors. If the child had experienced an electric shock, the picture, presentation and aftermath would have been completely different.

Electric current can surprise a person, produce pain and lead to a variety of events, including involuntary muscular contractions, spasms and resultant movements. There is typically a scream. The body may be thrown and it may jerk. There is often strong muscle contraction from nerve or muscle stimulation. Startle, neural, reflex and muscular reactions can result in serious injuries in persons who have received an electric shock. If electrocuted at height, they may fall and sustain an acute vertical deceleration injury.

In summary, I was not convinced that this child had sustained an electric shock. The finding in this case was more in keeping with that of an epileptic attack.

Cases of electrocution are typically complex, and an expert in the field, such as an independent electrical engineer, a municipal electrical engineer or an authority from a contracted academic institution, should be called to the scene to record the case for scientific and legislative purposes. Often, it will be difficult for a medical person to understand what precisely happened from an electrical point of view, while the converse is also possible and the electrical engineer may have difficulty understanding the medical perspective, so good communication should be established. Both parties should endeavour to simplify their explanations as much as possible so as that they (and the courts) can understand them.

In the case of a fatal electrical incident, a thorough post-mortem examination is performed taking Locard's Exchange Principle into account. Special attention must be paid to the clothing and shoes as these might display irregularities and must therefore be saved as physical evidence. It should be specifically determined if the victim was wet, dry or covered in sweat at the time of the incident. Notes must be made of any evidence of resuscitation attempts; specifically, any signs of defibrillation paddle marks.

Metal objects may have burned the underlying skin or may have been marked by the heat of electrical arcing. Metallic objects such as jewellery, tooth fillings, spectacles, a belt, buckles, coins and pacemakers should be specifically commented upon.

A meticulous description of the electrical burn wound should be made, with reference to its appearance and position on the body. The type, pattern and distribution of any cutaneous electrothermal injuries – in other words, electricity-induced skin injuries – should be documented. Electrocution entrance and exit wounds need to be commented upon. Particular attention must be paid to any grounding injuries (where the current exits the body), which may help reconstruct the position of the victim at the time of electrocution.

The possible current pathway through the body should be noted (e.g., through the chest, head, etc). Seek out signs of arc-blast – this is when electrical devices may explode and cause barotrauma injury, which results from changes in barometric (air) pressure. Examine the victim for rupture of eardrums. Check for singed and/or scorched hair and eye damage, such as retinal detachment. If the person electro-cuted was working on a roof, ladder or pole, additional fall-related blunt force injuries may be seen. Seek out fractures and amputations.

The procedure for internal examination is identical to that of any careful forensic autopsy. Specific attention should be paid to the presence or absence of electrical petechiae (pin-point haemorrhages typically found in the fissures of the lungs). Seek out electronic devices within the body, such as implantable cardioverter-defibrillators (used to treat tachy-arrhythmias or abnormal heart rhythms), which can cause an electrical discharge of 25 to 40 joules and may acciden-tally shock the pathologist. If such a device is found, the procedure should commence carefully. Manufacturers of the devices should be contacted as they typically have service representatives with deactivation processes.

The point of contact on the body surface with the electri-cal source may, through Locard's Exchange Principle, have skin lesions, which are called either electrical burns or elec-trical marks (although the term 'joule burn' is now gaining popularity). These are the sites of entry of the current. Other marks may appear where the body was earthed or grounded (grounding injuries). Fatal electrocution may appear with no skin marks and non-fatal electrocution may occur with skin marks. The skin mark usually has the appearance of a col-lapsed blister with raised edges and a pale areola. Histology of the skin mark is not always 100 per cent pathognomonic of an electrothermal event, and diagnosis based on a sin-gular skin lesion is often extremely difficult.

Interestingly, when it comes to high-voltage electrocution, contact is not necessarily required. Sometimes you can be electrocuted from about 35 cm away from a high-voltage source. Sparks literally jump the air gap and dance on the surface of your skin, creating a 'crocodile skin' injury pattern. This is one of the few examples where absolute contact is not necessary and yet the victim will still be overcome and possibly die.

In the instance of an electrocution event, there may or may not be a fresh burn mark on the skin. The formation of a fused nodule of keratin would require the tissues directly under the contact point to have reached a temperature of about 95 degrees centigrade. Tissue damage occurs within 25 seconds when the temperature reaches a mere 50 degrees centigrade. Remember that wounding depends on the time, nature and intensity of contact.

It is important to note that not all burn-appearing injuries are due to electrocution. Sepsis, drug reactions and heat are just a few electrocution injury mimics. Finally, any underlying risk factors in the victim of the electrocution should be excluded, such as, say, an underlying heart disease or possible epilepsy. The heart and brain should be carefully examined in the fresh state or after formalin fixation if an abnormality is seen or suspected.

The bathroom is a common site for electrical tragedies. In one instance, the naked bodies of a 25-year-old woman and her three-year-old son were found in a bathtub in their home. This incident happened in August 2018 – winter in South

Africa. An electric metal urn, containing minimal water, was connected to a plug point inside the bathroom. Apparently, it fell into the tub.

Autopsies were performed the following day. The female body showed electrothermal contact-burn wounds on the right side of the face and the right upper and left lower limbs. The body of the male child showed an electrothermal burn wound on the right foot. Locard's Exchange Principle helped recreate the scene. The urn had touched the right foot of the young boy. The current had passed through both bodies and exited through the mother's body, where she was in contact with the chrome taps.

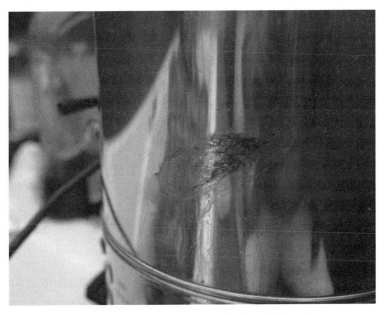

This mark on the metal urn is proof of electrical contact.

This case was unique in that it represented a double death due to electrocution in a bathtub.[1]

As a forensic pathologist, I have even been called upon to deliver testimony in cases of electrocution torture.

In June 2013, a 52-year-old man was discovered murdered, his wrists tightly ligated behind his back with wire and his ankles bound with a black belt. Due to the sensitivity of the case, I cannot supply further details about the circumstances under which he was found.

The man's conjunctivae were congested and a petechial haemorrhage was noted within the left eye. There were blunt force trauma injuries to the face, upper arms, left inguinal region, left inner thigh and sole of the left foot.

Two atypical skin injuries were noted on the chest wall. A bloodless field dissection of the neck showed discrete intramuscular haemorrhages. Two large subpleural blood-filled bullous lesions were noted on the lungs underlying the two atypical skin injuries on the chest wall. (The pleura is a thin layer of tissue that covers the lungs and lines the interior wall of the chest cavity.)

The claim of possible electrical abuse was raised in court and electrical torture was not contested. Three suspects were arrested and are currently serving time in prison for murder.

In instances of electrical torture, various devices have been used, ranging from metal bedframes to modified cattle prods. The *picana* or *picana eléctrica* is a device used to give an electric shock during electrical torture. It is a wand or prod that delivers a high-voltage, low-current, electric shock to torture victims. The current may be applied anywhere, although the genitals are a site favoured by torturers, especially the penis and the scrotum. The female nipples are also favoured targets. Atypical skin injuries may be seen in such cases.

In 2008 I was once again contacted by a human rights attorney who litigates torture cases. A prison inmate alleged that warders had used water in conjunction with an electro-shocking device to inflict and maximise physical and psychological pain on him. The question arose as to the effect that dousing a victim with water would have in exacerbating the shock experienced by that victim. A force-electrified riot shield was apparently used to torture the inmate.

I was asked to give an idea of the strength of the shock experienced so that a layman might understand. I was also asked to provide an idea of what would happen if the victim were either wet or dry. Would there be a difference between normal tap water and pure water, and which would be the better conductor? Would there be a difference if the energy output was constant and not pulsed? These were the kinds of questions and challenges posed to me with regard to the claim of possible electrical abuse. (My answers are beyond the scope of this book.)

There was another case of interest too. One morning in May 2013, a 30-year-old man was arrested, after which he was questioned by the police and officially booked into the cells. I cannot recall what crime he was suspected of. He was booked out for a confession to be taken from him. On his return, no injuries were noted down.

In court, the defence objected to the admissibility of his confession on the grounds that, inter alia, the accused had been assaulted. No details of an assault were given. However, a witness testified that she had heard that the accused had been electrocuted in the region of his private parts. On the morning of his first appearance in court there was a report of a fresh wound, the size of a 50-cent coin, on his genitals. The defence also submitted a blood report drawn a day later. I was consulted as an expert to examine the wound for signs of possible electrocution. Suffice to say, many textbooks have been filled with lists of the diseases that can cause a 50-cent-sized wound on the genitals. As you can imagine, my findings were inconclusive.

As can be seen, electrocution can happen in a variety of ways. Some are fatal, whereas some are not. The scenarios may be any of the following and many more: a person is found dead next to an electric iron, or in the bath with a hairdryer. Many have died while tampering with an electrical box, illegally connecting electrical wiring or after sticking their fingers into a live electrical socket. There has even been a case of a child who was found lifeless after biting into an electrical wire and a person who was heard screaming as they opened the fridge door and then collapsed dead.

A timely and thorough scene investigation is critical, especially where few or no physical findings at autopsy are present.

Paramount to scene investigation is safety: first and foremost, the scene should be made safe, as live electric wires would pose a threat to emergency personnel, police service officers, detectives and others engaged with an investigation. The mains have to be switched off. Care must be taken to ensure that the scene and body are not still electrified. Those on the scene must verify that the electricity has been turned off: double-check, triple-check, quadruple-check! The electrocution of paramedics and forensic investigators on the scene can be both tragic and quite embarrassing.

In informal settlements, there may be illicit connections that are often removed by residents before the police arrive at the death scene. In the instance of a defective device, the device itself may be the only evidence of electrocution after a thorough investigation and examination. Any electrical devices associated with the deceased must therefore be secured and forensically examined.

The wirings inside electrical devices consist of three main parts: the live wire, the neutral wire, and the earth wire. The live wire delivers the power supply to the device, while the neutral wire sends back the current received from the power supply to complete the circuit. The earth wire's role is protection. It is crucial to differentiate between the wires for safety purposes. Therefore each of the three wires has a specific, coloured insulator. The live wire is insulated using a brown plastic covering, the neutral wire using a blue plastic covering, and the earth wire using a green and yellow striped plastic covering.

Although safety measures are taken into consideration when electrical devices are being designed, faults can still occur due to a failure in installation or an insulation bridging. If the earth wire is missing in the event of a fault, the current will take an alternate path to the ground. If the body contacts the live wire, the current can enter and exit the body, leading to electrocution if the current is high enough. This is why the presence of the earth wire is crucial.[2]

On a more personal note, in April 2010 I was called to the tragic scene where a luxury train had derailed between Centurion and Pretoria. Sixteen of the carriages crashed into each other and others were overturned when the accident happened. Some of the carriages landed on passengers. The scene was chaotic with bodies strewn everywhere. A spokesperson for the emergency medical care provider ER24 said at the time: 'Some of the passengers were thrown from the carriages and others were trapped inside. Most of the injured people sustained multiple bone fractures.'[3]

In total, 25 tourists and some of the train's personnel were admitted in a serious condition to various hospitals in Pretoria and Johannesburg. Three people, one of whom was a pregnant woman, died in the accident. Naturally, there were live electrical wires everywhere. It was necessary to secure the site as quickly as possible to prevent any further loss of life or injury. What makes this accident so hard for me to forget is that people looted the train carriages immediately after the crash and stole bottles of wine and other items, disregarding the dead and injured, and amidst all the hazardous live electrical wires.

CASE STUDY 1

In December 2004, at approximately 16:00, a young child got stuck under an electric fence and died on a farm in the Western Cape. B was 12 years old at the time of the incident and lived on the farm.

As there was no water available at their house, a group of boys planned to get water in a bucket from a nearby stream and had to pass beneath the fence, since there were no gates in the fence. After they got the water, they returned with the bucket. One of the boys went first, then the next, and B went last. The other two held the bucket as B went under the fence. A wooden plank was present under the fence; however, B accidentally touched the electric wire and began to shake, going red in the face.

The boys ran back get help. At the scene, B was lying on his right side with his face in the water and his feet in the stream. When his father arrived, he tried to pull the child away from the fence and he too was shocked.

An ambulance was called, which took B to the local day hospital. Mouth-to-mouth resuscitation was performed the entire time. Tragically, the boy was declared dead on arrival. A sergeant who had visited the scene of the incident noted that the electric fence surrounding the property displayed no warning sign to notify passers-by that it was electrified. B required a medico-legal autopsy, which was performed in the local jurisdiction. The cause of death was stated as electrocution.

CASE STUDY 2

I was once approached by attorneys representing a teenage boy who had been involved in an electrocution incident. Apparently, in 2018, when he was 12 years old, he and another child were exposed to 88-kilovolt lines in Johannesburg. He survived and was admitted to the local academic hospital and treated for electrical burn wounds to the right leg, which required a skin graft.

Six months later, he presented with a history of persistent vomiting after eating, as well as watery diarrhoea. Apparently, he was also suffering abdominal pain, and he was very malnourished. The attorneys wanted to establish if there could be a link between the abdominal problems and the electrocution.

At presentation, he was noted to be wasted and pale. There were small lymph nodes, submandibular and axillary. His weight was 22 kg and he was 1.38 metres tall. Examination showed a scaphoid-shaped abdomen, pigmented skin lesions were noted at places and he showed signs of malnutrition. An HIV test was negative. An abdominal sonar and gastroscopy were performed and he had a full TB work-up.

The clinical plan was to continue weight monitoring and nutritional rehabilitation. He continued to complain of abdominal pains and loss of appetite. Nine months later, he was noted as weighing 20.1 kg. He underwent rigid and flexible gastroscopy and biopsy, however, no significant findings were identified by the paediatric surgeon. He still complained of generalised abdominal pain and his weight remained at 20.1 kg.

To summarise, the young man had a normal gastroscopy, no auto-immune diseases, normal thyroid functions and no features of malrotation. TB was ruled out. No temperature spikes were observed during admission.

I reviewed the case and requested all the data. There seemed to be sufficient evidence to support a history of an electrothermal incident. 'Post electric shock syndrome'[4] has been proposed in electric shock survivors; however, it is relatively rare and is a diagnosis of exclusion. I told the attorneys that I had never ever read in the literature about chronic diarrhoea, vomiting or abdominal pain following an electrical event. To date, I am still not aware of any evidence in the literature to support this claim.

First and foremost, all underlying pathology needed to be excluded by a gastroenterologist. I suggested that all medical conditions first needed to be excluded. In other words, all organic pathology needed to be ruled out first. Arsenic poisoning, for example, may present with diarrhoea, vomiting and abdominal pain. Such is the differential diagnosis of chronic diarrhoea. All aetiologies must be excluded first.

In conclusion, in my opinion, there was no link between the abdominal problems and the electrocution.

CASE STUDY 3

In another case that was rather challenging, a person died after touching a garden appliance. During the autopsy, we noticed four small dot-like wounds, spaced approximately two centimetres apart on the dorsal aspect of their hand. The differential diagnosis was either snakebite or electrocution, however, no snake had been witnessed at the scene.

First, we consulted a local snake expert to get an idea of what kinds of snakes, whether local or international, could potentially have killed so quickly. The expert told us that the only indigenous snake that could have caused a sudden death like that would have been a black mamba. However, the distance between the puncture wounds was off by 33 per cent if the snake had bitten from the lateral aspect of the hand.

'That leaves two punctures from over the fingers which are then even at two centimetres apart, so the snake would have bitten from the finger side of the hand. Both sets of punctures were not deep wounds and the wounds looked too big for the fangs of a black mamba. Mambas do not chew, although for two bites one would expect to see some other teeth grazing the fingers. If one looks at the skull of a black mamba, one gets an idea of the distance between the fangs and the diameter of the fangs,' he said.

A photograph of a black mamba bite, where the snake was 2.1 metres in length, showed some surrounding ecchymosis (subcutaneous haemorrhages), which is not common.

Another snake considered by the snake expert was the snouted cobra, which is very common in the area where the victim lived. Snouted cobra venom is far weaker and asphyxia would only be expected after two to three hours.

One should always keep in mind that there are secret snake breeders and exotic pet enthusiasts with rare and wonderful species living among us. Another exotic snake that could reach the height of the garden appliance (80 cm to 1 m) would be the taipan. The genus *Oxyuranus* does not kill that quickly, although fatality within half-an-hour could be realistic, with a double bite; the problem is that there are very few in South Africa, so the chances of one escaping and surviving in that region would have been very slight. They have powerful procoagulant toxins which would have caused more severe wounds at the bite site. The neurotoxins produced by this genus are postsynaptic and not that rapid in onset.

According to the snake expert, the king cobra could also fit the bill, however, for one to rear up that high it would need to be 2.5 metres long (which is not impossible). They are shy and retiring snakes that would not just bite and leave. If they are angry enough to bite, they stay hooded for an extended period and the witnesses would surely have seen it.

The krait (*Bungarus* genus) possesses powerful neurotoxins which are predominantly painless, however, the venom is fairly slow-acting and death is very rare in less than one hour. 'Reaching [the height of the garden appliance] is unlikely due to the fact that they don't grow that big and are mostly nocturnal and will hide during the day. Even when disturbed, they are reluctant to bite. Most of the other large snakes which can cause death routinely have more cytotoxic venoms which would take longer and cause local tissue necrosis, which is missing from this scenario,' the expert said.

The four dots on the hand were never adequately explained. They could even have been there before the person's death. This led us, *via negativa*, to consider electrocution on the differential diagnosis. If a person has wet or sweaty hands, electrocution may leave no visible marks on the body.

Many electrical deaths are not observed and the person is only found dead later. Sometimes, the witnessed mode of death is hard to explain on physiological grounds alone, in that there appears to be a delay (often some minutes in duration) between the shock and the death. In the interval, the victim may be conscious and even appear to be recovering. It is difficult to know why a sudden cardiac arrest should take place after the current is switched off, presumably some fundamental damage has been caused on an intracellular level to cardiac or neural tissue.[5]

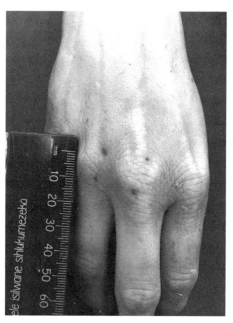

The only external injury noted on a person who died suddenly and unexpectedly.

9

Cause and effect – did this cause that?

So, you come down with the following symptoms at 15:00 on a Friday afternoon: headache, fever and gastroenteritis. All day you have been at your desk, except for the lunch that you bought from the vendor at the corner at 13:00.

Naturally, then, your provisional conclusion is that your symptoms are due to something you ate for lunch: that hot-dog, or the sauce . . . or perhaps it was the fish you had at dinner the previous night. You might even think you contracted Covid-19.

The last thing on your mind is the trip to the Kruger National Park – a malaria risk area – you took two weeks ago and that you might have contracted *Plasmodium falciparum* malaria, which has an incubation period of 21 days. This is another example of that informal fallacy of reasoning called *post hoc, ergo propter hoc* – after this, therefore because of this.

After a few years of Covid-19 we now know a bit more about cause and effect and how we come to conclude what the actual cause may be. I would like to discuss the virus and the

97

pandemic that changed our lives so dramatically from a forensic pathological perspective. I will stick to my field of expertise, and not discuss the virus itself, or the widespread effects of the pandemic on our physical, mental and emotional well-being.

The SARS-CoV-2 (severe acute respiratory syndrome coronavirus 2) pandemic wrought havoc on health-care systems around the world. (The name was chosen because the virus was genetically related to the coronavirus responsible for the SARS outbreak of 2003.) We were all faced with a new and dystopian reality. Trying to keep abreast of the latest literature on Covid-19 proved challenging indeed, causing doctors to sail uncharted oceans without their textbooks. Doctors were flooded with new information about a new virus. At the start of the pandemic, we were all out of our comfort zones, medical and non-medical colleagues alike. Adapting to *not* knowing was an important part of the learning process. Like everyone, many health-care workers suffered physically, psychologically and emotionally.

At the start of the pandemic I performed my first SARS-CoV-2 autopsy, then another, then another. Essentially, these were unnatural deaths with SARS-CoV-2 also present, for example a patient with Covid-19 (SARS-CoV-2) who died while undergoing a medical procedure. Or a person who had been in a motor vehicle accident who was SARS-CoV-2 positive. I also performed autopsies on sudden unexpected death cases which turned out to be SARS-CoV-2-positive.

Articles describing the known pathology and autopsy findings in SARS-CoV-2 soon began to circulate. There were recommendations for conducting autopsies in suspected SARS-

CoV-2 cases. There were suggested techniques for making the diagnosis at autopsy.[1] Adequate ventilation was required when performing such high-risk autopsies. These high-risk cases required 'enough separation' from the rest of the mortuary. Either whole-room ventilation or downdrafts at the workstation were advised.

Electric bone saws had to have a vacuum that isolated aerosolised particles. Bone dust from an oscillating headsaw was deemed deadly. Aerosol-generating procedures were not advised at such autopsies. We had to use manual bandsaws. SARS-CoV-2 was described as highly transmissive and one article showed that the virus had been isolated up to 35 hours post-mortem from the nasopharyngeal mucosa.[2]

All the while, the pandemic was hitting closer to home. I began losing family members and colleagues. The numbers were no longer statistics: they suddenly represented people that I knew.

'Am I burned out or infected?' became a common refrain.

Personally, I was inundated by messages and texts from everyone who had my phone number. This in itself nearly broke me. I was seriously at my limit. Every day I was receiving about twenty to thirty texts from family and friends asking me for my advice about the vaccines, about chloroquine, about ivermectin, and so on. I was literally getting hundreds of messages and phone calls asking for my opinion from everyone who had access to me. It really wore me down.

One good thing was that during the peaks of the different waves of the pandemic, each medical discipline added its own contributions to knowledge. Radiologists helped to decipher X-rays, palliative care experts brought their wealth of knowledge, and forensic pathologists were knee-deep in the mud, guts and blood of it all. Personal protective equipment became the norm. In clinical medicine, amidst all the chaos and uncertainty, the hierarchy of medicine seemed to fall away, thereby levelling the playing field: consultants, registrars, medical officers, interns and students worked side by side, doing whatever they could to help.[3]

Though it was uncharted territory, to me it felt very similar to our first HIV/AIDS autopsies, when the disease first broke out in the 1980s. (Yes, I was around then!)[4] The human immunodeficiency virus resulted in serophobia among staff working in mortuaries (i.e., a fear that any form of contact with HIV-infected patients or cadavers would lead to their infection). Yet there has been little evidence that HIV is readily acquired in the mortuary. HIV has been isolated from deceased persons with post-mortem intervals of 6, 11 and 16 days. HIV remains viable in the spleen at room temperature for at least 14 days. Outside the body, the virus is not hardy, and is inactivated by drying and by several disinfectants.

Lockdown exposed weaknesses in the human condition. Isolation was not healthy for our communal human spirit. After all, we humans are social creatures. We could not escape and we were all effectively under some kind of house arrest. Many people lost their jobs and many others worked from home. The pandemic almost completely decimated the restaurant, entertainment and tourism industries. It made us rethink how we did things and highlighted both our strengths and our weaknesses. Corruption seemed to rear its ugly head. The pandemic even made us question our experts.

'Who is the person giving us this advice?'

'Can we trust this expert?' we wondered.

They say a watched pot never boils. Well, it is my belief that an unwatched human typically does boil. People tend to become troublesome if there is no one to watch over them. Corporate culture was the first to suffer, because people were working from home and there was often no one to watch over or peer-review their colleagues. People were now living in their own 'mental vaults' without doors or windows. It was little surprise that I started seeing more corporate people on my autopsy table. (I could clearly see the effects of Locard's Exchange Principle: I was witnessing the consequences of 'contact' and the consequences of 'no contact'. I was seeing a change in people's behaviour, their patterns of living, and the consequences thereof.)

There was some good which came out of the pandemic too: industries like online shopping and online entertainment thrived, and working from home showed us that we were capable of some very innovative solutions, like online plat-forms. We also had time to catch up with ourselves. Time to reflect. Nature had time to revive. Birds moved into areas where they had never lived before, and, with lockdown, birds sang softer because there was less noise pollution.

Eventually we emerged from our lockdowns and were able to socialise again. We gave each other earnest verbal greet-ings and there was an unspoken kinship that we now all share. We welcomed each other back to our communities with sincerity. We all have our own Covid-19 war wounds. Hopefully, we are finally entering the home stretch and can all resume business as usual. However, as one of my colleagues succinctly put it, we are seeing the light at the end of the tunnel, but we just don't know how long the tunnel is.

What were the effects of lockdown-implemented restrictions like curfews, alcohol bans and cigarette bans on our forensic pathology workload in South Africa? There were five trends that I noticed, subjectively, from my autopsy table.

First, there seemed to be an increase in suicides. On my autopsy table I was seeing chiefly corporate people: lawyers, bankers and businesspeople who had committed suicide. Catastrophic financial problems and worry appeared to be the most likely cause. People's mental health was definitely being affected. Quarantine and isolation requirements for the early victims of Covid-19 contributed largely to psychological instability, especially for those who could not contact their families or loved ones.[5] Not being able to socialise may also have had its consequences; isolation cannot be good for your mental health, especially if you are an extrovert. Children especially require socialisation to be well balanced in life.

Watching what was happening in old-age homes broke my heart. The elderly couldn't see their children or grandchildren, and they couldn't even play bingo.

From the suicides that I was seeing, it appeared that hanging was the most common method. (This is probably the case because all that is needed is a rope and one's own body weight.) The youngest case of hanging I saw during the hard lockdown was that of a seven-year-old child.

Second, there seemed to be an increase in addiction-type deaths. Most likely, people were not getting their usual fixes and so they resorted to dangerous alternatives: methanol from home brews and impure illicit drugs seemed to be the order of the day. I performed an autopsy on a person who had made his own homemade whisky. Three of the deceased's friends also died from the same whisky brew.

A one-litre bottle of home-made alcohol-type beverage, labelled W, accompanied his body to the mortuary. What these home brewers did not realise was that the first batch of alcohol is usually poisonous – it is pure methanol.

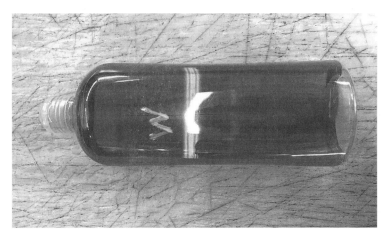

The deadly bottle of home-made alcohol.

During the distillation process methanol is concentrated at the start of the production run because it has a lower boiling point than ethanol (the good stuff) and water. The first compounds released in the still as it heats up are the lower-boiling-point compounds, which we call the heads or head product.[6] These compounds typically include methanol, acetaldehyde and lighter esters. You should never drink the heads of moonshine!

Home brewers may produce small quantities of methanol when they distil using commercial spirit yeasts and sugar or dextrose. Homemade spirits, such as moonshine, hooch and white dog, can easily be made the wrong way and then contain toxic methanol. Pure methanol may cause blindness and even kill you.

The rookie home brewer does not know how to remove methanol from their homebrew, however, a commercial distiller will typically discard methanol. Distilling alcohol at home can therefore present great risks.

Third, I was seeing an increase in interpersonal, partner-related violence. For people who were living together there was nowhere to run and nowhere to hide. Partners had to confront one another, face-to-face, and this sometimes ended in disaster.

Fourth, I started seeing a lot more transport-related deaths when lockdown restrictions were eased. The world was sent to their room, and what happens when someone is sent to their room for a long time? They tend to become angry. Also, their reflexes slow down. People seemed to forget how to drive properly, or perhaps their confidence levels dropped. There seemed to be an increase in road traffic fatalities. There was also a slight uptick in road rage cases.

Finally, I was seeing an increased number of skeletons

and decomposed bodies, simply because no one was finding all the lonely people in their rooms and flats and apartments. There were also fewer joggers finding dead bodies in the fields. (Joggers always seem to be the ones who first discover bodies in the outdoors.)

These days one cannot consider Covid-19 without discussing vaccines, however, before we do that, we need to understand some basic definitions. These definitions will help us better understand *if this really caused that.*

Let us take the following example: insurance companies have accidental death policies which require that *accidental deaths* be *accidental.* What do we write on the death certificate if a heart attack (a natural death) causes a motor vehicle accident (an unnatural death)? Or what happens if death results when epilepsy (a natural condition) causes a fall from a great height (an unnatural death)?

As mentioned before, if you are seeking to understand whether an event leading to death was contributed to or caused by the consumption of drugs or alcohol, what are the ultimate questions to ask in such a situation? Firstly, you always have to ask if a drug or poison was present or absent. What sort of action could the substance have exerted on the deceased? Was the drug present in sufficient quantity to affect the behaviour or well-being of the donor of the sample? Could the substance have influenced the person at the time of the alleged incident? These 'drugs on board' situations can be tricky.

In forensic pathology, we define the *primary* medical cause of death as the disease or injury which initiated the process or sequence of physiological events or complications which led to the death of the patient. In other words, it is the first domino in the entire Domino Rally (also known as Domino Express). The *terminal* cause of death is usually a complication that follows.

Take the example of a head injury with pneumonia. The head injury is the primary medical cause of death. The pneumonia is the terminal cause of death. What this means is that if a doctor sees a patient who died from pneumonia, that doctor may be tempted to certify the death as due to natural causes – whereas, in fact, that person could have been hit on the head with a brick several weeks beforehand, thus sustaining a head injury, been lying in hospital unresponsive, and ultimately died of the complication of pneumonia, because that person couldn't breathe or cough by themselves.

If the doctor signs the death certificate as 'natural causes' this victim will simply be buried or cremated and the murderer will walk free! If, however, the doctor realises that the pneumonia is a complication of the head injury, the doctor will certify the death as owing to unnatural causes and an inquest will be opened, which could help catch the brick-throwing murderer. The head injury is the primary medical cause of death, whereas the pneumonia is the terminal cause of death. We now have a clearer picture of the sequence of events and we now understand what happened first. Understanding cause and effect may be extremely difficult, because there may be additional factors that contribute to an earlier death.

Not understanding these basic definitions wreaked havoc when it came to writing death certificates during the Covid-19 pandemic. Many doctors and nurses were mistaking the terminal medical cause of death for the primary cause of death. A death certificate has two functions: an administrative function (to register the death, as a statutory requirement, and as a prerequisite for the family to wrap up the estate of the deceased) and a statistical function (details of the deceased and the cause of death being used to gather mortality statistics for the country).[7] Not understanding these basic definitions will severely affect a country's administrative and statistical functions. With this explained, I now want to discuss vaccination deaths.

Every day, people die from natural and unnatural causes. Statistically, some of these people will have received a vaccination shortly before their deaths. So, how many are bona fide vaccination deaths? (By the way, I am not an anti-vaxxer: I believe in vaccination because it saves lives, I have seen that. Yet make no mistake, there are vaccine-related deaths.) Ultimately, it is all about the health of the human herd. Veterinarians, for example, may lose one or two sheep due to vaccination; however, the herd itself will survive. Veterinarians call it 'herd health'.

The average person most likely doesn't know the difference between the words 'vaccination' and 'immunisation'. 'Vaccination' describes the process of receiving a vaccine; that is, actually getting the injection or taking an oral vaccine dose. 'Immunisation' refers to the whole process, both getting the vaccine and becoming immune to the disease following vaccination.

If a person receives a vaccination and dies immediately, that person will obviously require a medico-legal autopsy. So, too, if that person dies one, two, six or twenty-four hours after their vaccination and there seems to be causality or nexus. Now, what happens if a person dies 21 days, six months or even a year after their vaccination? Are these cases also vaccine-related deaths? Do these cases demand a thorough medico-legal examination? What is the cut-off period for a so-called vaccine-related death? What is happening in other countries around the world?

Forensic pathologists deal with patterns. We are experts at pattern recognition. As an example, we look at the pattern of injuries, and it is the pattern of injuries, not an individual injury, that is important. If someone dies 21 days after receiving a vaccination, is it due to the vaccine or due to something completely different? What happens if I find a deep venous thrombosis or pulmonary embolism or heart attack as the cause of death at autopsy? Would the sudden death have happened had the person not been vaccinated?

I know that this is an almost impossible question to answer. However, what happens if I start seeing many deaths due to deep venous thrombosis, or pulmonary embolisms, or heart attacks, 21 days after vaccination? In other words, what happens if I see a pattern develop? Then surely, my forensic brain must kick into action. The Paul-Ehrlich-Institut uses 30 days as a cut-off period for autopsy after vaccination because there have been reports of myocarditis (inflammation of the heart muscle) within 30 days of mRNA vaccination, as reported by the Israeli Ministry of Health.[8]

This also highlights the importance of the world working together, because what happens if I see a rare death, a colleague in the UK sees a similar rare death and a colleague in Australia sees a similar one? How would we all know about our respective rare deaths, unless there were excellent communication channels between us and excellent global data capturing? What I am talking about is real-time global communication. If pathologists do not speak with one another, rare deaths will go undocumented.

The same applies to serial killers, or weird and rare cancers. If we did not have platforms to alert our professional associates to such cases, the world would be a much more frightening place. Luckily, we have international journals, global registries and surveillance bulletins to help report adverse effects, outbreaks and rare phenomena.

This highlights the public health role of medical examiner offices.[9] Often the first presentation of a new disease is death. In other words, these people don't even make it to the emergency room; they come straight to the mortuary. Who else, other than your friendly pathologists, will be able to diagnose the weird and wonderful pathologies associated with Covid-19?[10]

10

Look to the environment

A 59-year-old male died suddenly at his home seven days after he had become aware of a bite of unknown origin on the back of his neck. He neither removed nor witnessed an insect on his neck. There was a report of a non-specific headache prior to his death. No other complaints were noted. It was suspected to be a spider bite, yet he did not seek medical help and no further medical records were available. The incident took place during the Covid-19 pandemic and it is unclear whether that may have deterred him from seeking medical assistance.

His body was referred for medico-legal investigation in accordance with South Africa's Inquests Act, Act 58 of 1959. The body was thin and showed poor or average nutrition (height 1.85 m; weight 80 kg). An eschar measuring 1.5 cm x 1.2 cm was found on the back of his neck. An eschar is a dry, dark scab or falling away of dead skin, typically caused by a burn, an insect bite or an infection with anthrax. The wound showed signs of healing.

Approximately 4 cm to the right of the eschar was an ulcer 0.5 cm in diameter (possibly another, smaller eschar – sometimes multiple bites are noted). Both wounds were excised for histological purposes. No further injuries or abnormalities to the body could be identified. There were multiple co-morbid factors present, such as background lung, heart and kidney disease. Examination of the blood vessels showed no obvious microthrombi (blood clots).

I immediately realised that this was not a case of a spider bite. It was more in keeping with a tick bite, because of the eschar. This prompted swift, specific investigations of other possible infectious causes of death. Post-mortem venous blood was sent to the laboratory for analysis and the results came back positive for *Rickettsia conorii*, which at the time of death supported my provisional diagnosis of tick bite fever.

In South Africa, tick bite fever is associated with either *R. conorii* or *R. africae*, infection with the former known to be associated with higher mortality and poorer clinical outcomes. The classical clinical triad for tick bite fever diagnosis is eschar, fever and rash, however, all three features are only found in approximately 50 per cent to 75 per cent of cases. My patient had no evidence of any rash, and no fever was reported.

R. conorii is mostly associated with dog and kennel ticks and is often reported in periurban or domestic locations in South Africa, and therefore exposure is plausible. Larvae or nymph stages of ticks may be missed due to their small size. It is not clear if the deceased felt the bite or discovered the eschar; it is unlikely that he would have been bitten only seven days prior to death, as the incubation period following a bite is typically five to seven days, and one would expect some clinical progression before death. Microscopic examination confirmed eschar formation. The absolute reason why he died remains elusive. The multiple co-morbid factors, plus the tick bite, together could possibly have contributed to his death.

Tick bite fever is a common cause of fever-based illness in South Africa and timely treatment with antibiotics such as doxycycline or chloramphenicol can be lifesaving.

Interestingly, several days after having performed the autopsy examination, I started feeling sick and developed joint pains and a headache. After all, I had entered the post-mortem thinking it was a spider bite and I was therefore somewhat relaxed with my personal protective equipment. I didn't predict that I would be dealing with a possible trans-

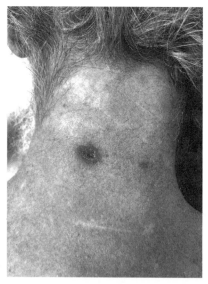

The eschar that was caused by a tick bite. Approximately 4 cm to the right of the eschar is an ulcer 0.5 cm in diameter (possibly another, smaller eschar – sometimes multiple tick bites are noted).

missible infectious disease. My own GP placed me on doxy-cycline and I lived to tell this tale.

On another note, I am not aware of any spiders that have killed people in South Africa. Yes, we do have some venomous ones in South Africa, although neither I nor any of my colleagues have performed an autopsy on a bona fide spider bite case within the borders of the country, according to my own knowledge at the time of writing.

By now, especially if you are South African, you will have realised that there are indeed many ways in which nature can be deadly.

I once did an autopsy on a man in his twenties who was admitted to an emergency room after sustaining envenomation (injection of venom into a person's body) from a black mamba (*Dendroaspis polylepis*). According to the available history, a single fang hooked his right index finger after he extracted venom from the snake. The victim remained in a coma for three days, after which he was declared dead.

A medico-legal post-mortem examination was performed four days after death. What made this matter so fascinating was that a single prick from a single fang of a black mamba had killed him. In my view, there was no way that enough venom could have been injected into the bloodstream through the tip of the index finger. How, then, did the black mamba venom manage to kill this young man? We all know that black mamba venom is venomous – yet, can it really be *that* venomous? Was there perhaps another mechanism at play?

There is minimal literature on the pathology of black

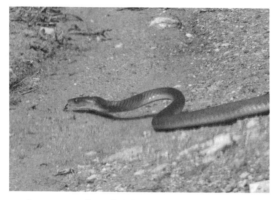

Black mambas are rarely truly black in colour. They are usually dark-brown, olive-brown or gunmetal. Photo: Karen Birkenbach

mamba bites. The black mamba is an elapid, with front fangs fixed to the upper jaw. It is a venomous snake, with neurotoxic venom, found in southern Africa. The mamba is born with approximately two to three drops of venom per fang (an adult having approximately 12–20 drops per fang). Only two drops of venom are required to kill an adult human. Of all venomous snakes in Africa, it is the largest and most feared. Most attacks happen during the mating season, spring or early summer, when it is more irritable and aggressive than usual.

As an example of the lethal potentialities of the mamba, one can quote the many cases when one of these snakes has been flushed out by a pack of inexperienced dogs, and four or more of the dogs have been bitten in rapid succession and subsequently succumbed before the snake could be torn to pieces. Although this snake has a reputation as being one of the most dangerous snakes in Africa, it tends to be shy and elusive and therefore avoids humans.

Returning to the case with the young man who had been bitten on the finger: he was accompanied by co-workers who were able to supply valuable information to the emergency room personnel on duty. It was reported that the victim worked as a snake handler in a facility where venomous snakes were milked for their venom to produce snake anti-venom. The victim had apparently finished milking a black mamba. (The co-workers were certain that the snake was a black mamba.)

After safely securing the snake in its cage, the man apparently walked over to a washbasin and proceeded to wash his hands. He then walked over to his colleague and reported that he felt dizzy and that he thought the snake might have bitten him when he released it into its cage. According to one co-worker, the victim was holding his right hand and was bleeding from the index finger.

Emergency measures were instituted by his co-worker, who placed a blood pressure cuff around the arm to stop the venom from entering the circulation, and he was immediately taken to the nearest hospital. The victim said he was feeling faint and was reported to be rubbing his lips over one another. They called ahead to the accident and emergency department to inform them that they were rushing a snakebite victim to hospital and that they would likely require antivenom.

The hospital pharmacy prepared all available antivenom and acquired more in case the need should arise. (Also known as antivenin, venom antiserum and antivenom immuno-globulin, it is a specific treatment for envenomation. It is composed of antibodies and used to treat certain venomous bites and stings. Antivenoms are recommended only if there is significant toxicity or a high risk of toxicity.)

The emergency doctors and personnel assessed the patient on arrival. Finding no pulse or spontaneous breathing, they commenced with immediate cardiopulmonary resuscitation, which comprised endotracheal intubation (a breathing tube placed into the windpipe), manual ventilation with high-flow 100 per cent oxygen and manual chest compressions. Intravenous access was obtained to administer fluids and inotropic support (allowing his heart to pump with more power). Shortly after cardiopulmonary resuscitation was commenced, a very feeble heart rate was recorded, with no regular rhythm returning.

The accident and emergency department doctor then consulted the extracorporeal membrane oxygenation (ECMO) team of the hospital to consider the patient for ECMO. Also known as extracorporeal life support, ECMO is a technique of providing prolonged cardiac and respiratory support to persons whose heart and lungs are unable to provide an adequate amount of gaseous exchange or perfusion to sustain life. ECMO is fast becoming part of the armamentarium (latest weaponry) for the physician treating catastrophic life-threatening emergencies.

The first 12 hours were critical in stabilising all parameters, and constant vigilance was applied to maintain all systems. Neurological assessment was acquired less than 24 hours after admission. The results were not promising. The patient's peripheral resistance remained low and adequate circulation could only be maintained through high dosages of peripheral vasoconstrictors, resulting in a steady low perfusion state and severe compounding metabolic acidosis. No neurological activity could be recorded on electrocardiography, and maintaining his circulation became increasingly difficult. No further escalation in treatment was possible and all cardiac activity ceased 72 hours after admission to the hospital.

External examination showed an adult male with a single puncture mark located approximately 0.5 cm from the fingernail on the lateral aspect of the right index finger. No obvious swelling could be seen in relation to the wound. Surrounding subcutaneous haemorrhage was present, which measured approximately 1 cm in diameter.

At autopsy, the body showed signs consistent with prolonged hospitalisation, multiple organ failure and disseminated intravascular coagulation. In other words there were a lot of haemorrhages within the body. The bladder contained approximately 20 ml of bloodstained urine. Histology of the fang puncture mark on the finger confirmed vital reaction, with associated haemorrhage noted at the skin puncture site. There was minimal skin necrosis at the bite mark. It was unlikely that the snake had injected a large amount of venom into an index finger, which puzzled me as to the reason why this young man had died.

Discussion with an international expert on snake venoms made me rethink the reason why this young man had died so quickly. An expert from Australia said this: 'I have no doubt that anaphylaxis contributed towards the fatal out-

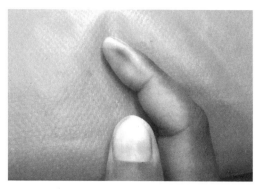

This single puncture mark was the only sign that
a snake handler had been bitten by a black mamba.

come. When one looks at the victim's profession, venom extractor/maintaining a large collection of venomous snakes etc., one must question the possibility and probability that he had developed a venom hypersensitivity through direct exposure over a period of time.

'Venom that has just been extracted and is still in its liquid form is stable and the probability of being exposed is low. However, this individual, along with his colleagues, stabilises the venom via "freeze drying". This then lyophilised [freeze-dried] product has a great potential of becoming an airborne antigen, and via nasal mucosa and/or ocular absorption, an individual can then become sensitised to this antigen, even developing an IgE Type-I response.

'The act of cleaning the enclosures also exposes the individual to venom. Venomous snakes will often express venom during feeding, when agitated, with spitting cobras being on the extreme end of that scale. Venom will dry in the cage substrate or the sides/glass front of the enclosure. Removing substrate/cleaning etc. can cause the dried venom to become airborne, again exposing the potential victim to the risks of becoming sensitised.

'I believe one or two of these exposures could well have triggered an immune sensitisation response. Based on the history of the events, the sudden collapse within minutes of being bitten, loss of consciousness and, eventually, prehospital cardiac arrest, the young man had become highly sensitised to *D. polylepis* (black mamba) venom and developed an immediate IgE mediated Type-I immune response.'

An acute allergic reaction to an antigen is called anaphylaxis. It is well known that such reactions can be serious. In this case, an urticarial rash was noted at ER which probably was related to anaphylaxis.

Upon review of this case, it is believed that this young man arrived at the hospital after having suffered cardiac arrest with accompanying hypoxic brain injury. The initial injury (the primary medical cause of death) – the fang prick envenomation by the black mamba – apparently put all events in motion which contributed to multiple organ failure in a very short period. (The act of cleaning snake enclosures probably exposed him to airborne antigen. The dried venom likely became airborne and attached to his mucosa, exposing and sensitising his immune system. The sudden (re)exposure in the form of the single fang bite to the index finger probably caused him to have a massive anaphylactic reaction).

Nature has a range of other 'killing methods', a common one being asphyxia. Sometimes there may be no external signs on the body, however, the circumstances suggest the cause. For example, a lover of exotic animals died of asphyxia after his 2.4-metre pet African rock python wrapped itself around him. The deceased was found dead by his mother, in his bedroom, with the python close by. There were ten pet snakes and 12 pet tarantulas in his bedroom at the time.

A post-mortem found that the deceased's lungs were four times heavier than would be expected and he had suffered pinpoint haemorrhages in one of his eyes: signs of asphyxia. He also had a freshly fractured rib. The forensic pathologist said: 'It's possible that some sort of pressure was applied to the neck or chest that caused him to asphyxiate.' However, there were no marks around his neck or chest.[1]

The big cats – lions and leopards – tend to like the neck. When you watch big cats kill antelope, you will note that they generally go for the neck. Packs of dogs tend to eat their prey alive, dismemberment with sharp teeth being their preferred method. The prey usually dies from exsanguination or shock. I have had several cases of victims being mauled by a pack of domestic dogs. In one such case, we managed to determine which specific dogs of the pack had done the mauling (and the eating). We did this by means of individualisation of the dog bite marks.[2] Dog bite marks can be matched to a relatively high degree of certainty.

This was a special application of Locard's Exchange Principle: if there are multiple points of concordance between the bite marks on the victim and the dentition of the suspected dog, the conclusion of a match with a high degree of certainty or high probability can be reached. Often a forensic expert may be required to identify which specific dog caused the injury or fatal bite to establish the identity of the owner or controller of the animal.[3]

Dogs are still wolves beneath their skin, and by owning a dog, any dog, humans welcome into their home a beast that preserves much of its primordial self. Like wolves, dogs attack the weak, be they young, old or drunk.[4] Seventy per cent of fatal dog-bite attacks are committed by a pet dog within the owner's yard or its proximity.[5]

As for marine deaths, it is important to understand the forensic pathology of noxious marine animals: sea snakes, sharks, cone shells, sea anemones, sea urchins, electric fish; all of these can injure and kill.

One of the most unusual killing methods employed by nature involves electricity. The electric eel (*Electrophorus electricus*) is a type of knifefish that can shock and stun its prey. It can generate powerful electric shocks of up to 600 volts which it uses for both hunting and self-defence. It is an apex predator in its South American range; however, there are a few specimens in South African aquariums.

The electric eel is unique in having large electric organs capable of producing lethal discharges that allow it to stun prey. It has three abdominal pairs of organs that produce electricity: the main organ, the Hunter's organ and the Sach's organ. These organs make up four-fifths of its body and are what give the electric eel the ability to generate two types of electric organ discharges: low voltage and high voltage. These organs are made of electrocytes, lined up so that the current flows through them and produces an electrical charge, in a manner similar to a battery, in which stacked plates produce an electrical charge.

Electric eels can vary the intensity of the electrical discharge, using lower discharges for hunting and higher intensities for stunning prey or defending themselves. When agitated, they are capable of producing intermittent electrical shocks over a period of at least an hour without signs of tiring. Electric eels are unlikely to cause a damaging electric shock to humans, although a shock from an electric eel would be an unpleasant experience. Signs explicable according to the Locard Exchange Principle on the body of someone exposed to an electric fish are almost impossible to observe.

CASE STUDY 1

I once examined the body of a young male who was believed to have been assaulted several days before death. I consulted forensic odontologists regarding the identification of the individual. I also requested an opinion on a suspected white bite mark on the left shoulder of the deceased. The general impression, shape and size of the mark were consistent with those of a human bite mark. There was macroscopic evidence of scab formation that indicated that it had been inflicted some time before death. In other words, there were macroscopic signs suggestive of wound healing.

Fresh wounds have medico-legal significance. Healing, and healed wounds, may also have medico-legal significance. I thought that the healing bite mark may therefore also be of value to the forensic investigation. The ageing and dating of bite marks are controversial, and there were no universally acceptable guidelines available to accurately predict this complex process.

The concept of wound ageing may be defined in terms of the time interval that exists between the infliction of the injury and the time of death. The process of tissue healing and tissue repair commences immediately after a wound is inflicted. When inflicted before death, the question often arises: how long before death was it sustained? Careful examination of skin wounds is essential in forensic pathology and is usually performed to ascertain wound age in relation to time of death.

Since the 1960s, the development of forensic histopathology has helped us with the estimated age of wounds. Patterned abrasions and intradermal bruises retain the pattern of the impacting object relatively accurately. In other words, Locard's Exchange Principle works with fresh wounds, healing wounds and (sometimes) even healed wounds. A careful examination of the skin may show the relatively well-preserved imprint of the impacting object – in this case, the teeth of the suspect.

Patterned injuries occur when a force is applied at or near a right angle to the skin surface. This scarred bite mark clearly showed histological time-associated processes, indicative of a prolonged time interval.

Skin is capable of healing when injured. The repair process leaves tell-tale signs at both the macroscopic (visual) and microscopic (histological, histochemical and biochemical) levels. Bite marks may vary from skin indentations with associated bruising to abrasions and to lacerated open wounds.

Ours was one of the first documented case reports in the literature of ageing a healing bite mark. In our case, we could prove that the bite mark on the left shoulder was at least seven to eight days old. Locard's Exchange Principle provided us with the only evidence connecting a particular suspect to our victim.[6]

We also have experience with bite marks on humans from animals, such as dogs. Dog bite marks, although similar to human bite marks in certain respects, need a modified analysis technique to accommodate the anatomical differences which exist in the canine dentition. We developed a relatively new technique to analyse and individualise a dog bite mark on a human being.[7]

———————

11

Weapons and Locard's Exchange Principle

I once had to deal with a case of a man who was found in the outdoors, dead next to his motorbike, with his helmet still on his head. Initially, it looked like a stock-standard motorbike accident and his body was removed for autopsy.

Luckily, we always X-ray the bodies before autopsy. What we found was quite astonishing: this wasn't the accident we had initially thought it was: multiple small pellets, together with a shotgun wad, were present in the deceased's intracranial cavity, inside his motorcycle helmet. Multiple fractures of the facial bones and calvaria (top part of the skull) could also be observed. There was a shotgun entrance wound within the oral cavity and the pellets appeared to have travelled from below to above, and from right to left.

It turns out that this was a very considerate person who committed suicide and didn't want to damage his surroundings with brain tissue and shotgun pellets. The man shot himself in the mouth, outdoors, with his motorcycle helmet on. The actual shotgun was only discovered later under his bike, when the bike was towed away.

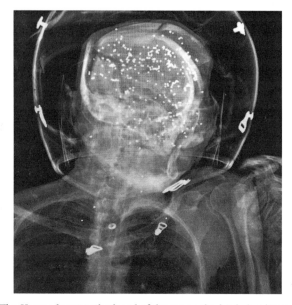

The X-ray showing the head of the man who had shot himself with his motorbike helmet on. He had shot himself through the mouth.

Forensic pathologists need to know a great deal about novel killing methods. One of our mandates as medical professionals is to help diagnose, and we must keep abreast of the latest information internationally. (To use movie parlance, we need to know what is 'coming soon to a mortuary suite near you'.) For this, forensic pathologists have scientific journals, which are an excellent source of new knowledge.

Sometimes we come across a weapon, or a technique, which we have never seen before. Locard's Exchange Principle can help diagnose even the most advanced killing methods.

There are four different scenarios when it comes to weapons and techniques:

- An old weapon using an old technique: In other words, the weapon is being used in the usual, old-fashioned way. Classic weapons are a knife and a gun.

- An old or classic weapon built using a new technique: For example, I have seen shotguns made from steel pipes and rubber bands, and empty shotgun shells filled with birdseeds, salt, sugar, sand or even cyanide powder.

- A new weapon used with an old technique: Imagine a modern handgun being used to knock someone over the head, because there were no projectiles present. In such an instance a relatively new weapon is being used like a baton, an ancient weapon, to cause blunt force head trauma.

- A new weapon using a new technique: This is probably the scariest technique, since it is a combination that could fool any forensic pathologist. The wound would probably be something new and puzzling that has been unheard of until now. An example of this would be if someone figured out how to weaponise lightning, for example. Imagine being able to control lightning or being able to cause lightning to strike at a specific place, for example at a weapon storage depot. This is not entirely impossible. If we can already generate lightning strikes by means of rocket triggering, then surely, we as humans have the capability to induce lightning strikes at will?

Using ultra-low-frequency sound as a weapon is another scary possibility. All objects resonate at certain

127

frequencies. What would happen if there were a sound-producing machine that resonates at the same frequency as your liver or your spleen, for example? We have seen a wine glass shatter at certain frequencies, far away from the source. What stops the development of a weapon that, from far away, can cause a liver or a spleen to rupture at a certain frequency?

These and many other such deadly techniques lurk in the murky underworld. We as forensic pathologists must be constantly vigilant for such things. We need to keep our ears to the ground and our eyes on the horizon, for it will probably be a forensic pathologist who first diagnoses such a new weapon's existence.

There are many different terrifying weapons, and over the years I have performed autopsies on hand grenade and shotgun cases, for example. I will never forget these cases, and consequently, as far as I am concerned, hand grenades and shotguns should be banned outright.

One of the scariest new forms of ammunition is the G2 RIP, otherwise known as the Radically Invasive Projectile. A G2 RIP round is one of the latest in a range of fragmenting and frangible projectiles. Because of the bullet's unique design, the wounds demonstrate characteristic radiographic patterns and present unique autopsy findings. It is designed to create massive wounding and rapid victim incapacitation.

The lead-free G2 RIP bullet is made of solid copper, which is machined into a base and up to eight fragments (referred to by the manufacturer as 'trocars') with pointed tips. The G2 RIP is therefore designed to produce large amounts of tissue damage. At autopsy, one typically finds multiple clusters and occasional, isolated, radio-opaque fragments. Trocars and the bullet base (the round fragment at the centre) may be recovered from victims. One needs to be very careful of the pointed tips of the trocars, which pose a safety hazard during projectile recovery. These trocars can easily penetrate the thickest of gloves given their sharpness, which poses a risk to the person doing the autopsy and other support personnel.

The trocars' trajectories disperse away from the central trajectory of the base, and they together create multiple wound channels. Recognising the radiograph patterns of the G2 RIP and familiarising yourself with the nature of the bullet fragments are important for both forensic pathologists and clinicians in procedure planning, projectile identification, projectile recovery, case documentation and personal safety. Not having read about such a projectile would leave the average doctor in the dark. When in doubt, a forensic pathologist must simply describe and document what they see. There are always other experts in the world able to help identify what has been observed.[1]

In forensic pathology, one differentiates between penetrating and perforating wounds. A penetrating wound means the object may go into or through something, although it doesn't necessarily emerge on the other side. In other words, there is no exit wound.

A perforating wound, by contrast, is an injury caused by an object which enters the body and passes through it. It is associated with an entrance wound *and an exit wound.*

In a multiple shooting case, if there are an even number of entrance and exit gunshot holes in the skin, it is likely that the projectiles went in and then out of the body; in other words, the body sustained perforating gunshot wounds, and there will be no projectiles retained within the body. If, however, there are an odd number of entrance and exit gunshot holes, it is likely that retained projectiles remain within the body.

Allow me to introduce a phenomenon that has fooled many a forensic pathologist. Imagine that a single gunshot entrance wound has been sustained and there is no gunshot exit wound – in other words, there is a penetrating gunshot entrance wound – however, after meticulous X-ray examination and a thorough autopsy examination, no projectile is discovered within the body or clothing. This phenomenon is termed 'vanishing projectile syndrome'.

It is hard to believe, but there are at least eight scenarios where this very real phenomenon may occur.

1. The projectile may strike a bone and then bounce (ricochet) out of the body.
2. The projectile may exit through the mouth, nostril, ear, vagina or rectum.
3. The projectile may be coughed, vomited or defecated out of the body.
4. The weapon may be a crossbow. (A site where a penetrating crossbow bolt has been manually removed

looks exactly like a gunshot entrance wound – it is a gunshot entrance wound mimicker – and no projectile will be found within the body.

5. The projectile may enter the aorta (the largest blood vessel in the body), and it may embolise to the most distal part of the leg or foot. The feet are often 'cut off' in whole-body X-rays, and the projectile may be missed.

6. Bismuth iodoform paraffin paste (BIPP) gauze is an antiseptic dressing that is typically used in acute epistaxis to stop nosebleeds. A crumpled-up piece of BIPP gauze in the nasal cavity looks exactly like a malformed projectile when viewed on X-ray and has fooled many a forensic pathologist.

7. A projectile may enter, exit, re-enter, re-exit, re-re-enter and re-re-exit the body. Often these wounds are atypical and can fool a forensic pathologist into thinking that there are more entrance gunshot wounds than exit gunshot wounds. The entrance and exit wounds might add up to an odd number, and you may suspect a projectile within the body, whereas in fact, there are no projectiles, because you misdiagnosed the gunshot wounds.

8. An old projectile may remain within the body from a previous penetrating shooting incident. This projectile confuses the forensic pathologist, especially in multiple gunshot wound cases. The extra projectile in the body can make one erroneously consider a variant of vanishing projectile syndrome.

In my own case files, I have an example of vanishing projectile syndrome where an X-ray of a deceased man showed three projectiles lodged within his body. After a thorough (and frustrating) autopsy, it transpired that two of the projectiles were actually the two ends of the deceased's blue drawstring hoodie, which the victim was wearing at the time of X-ray examination! There was only one projectile in the body. Now that's a rookie mistake!

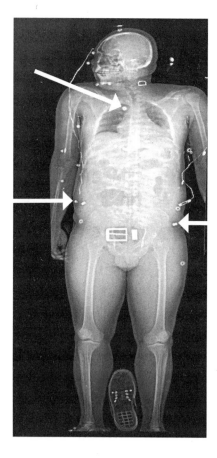

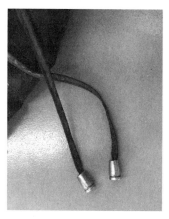

Left: *An X-ray of the victim seemed to indicate three projectiles within the body. The arrows on the right and left show the 'vanished' projectiles that I spent hours searching for. The arrow at the top shows the real projectile.*

Right: *The culprits: the drawstring ends of a hoodie that I had mistaken for projectiles!*

CASE STUDY 1

In June 2017, a 34-year-old male that I shall call Mr A arrived at a hospital casualty unit at 17:30. Apparently, he had sustained a gunshot wound to the left lower leg. It was alleged that he had been shot by a policeman while running away.

Dr J originally assessed and managed Mr A in the casualty unit. Her admission notes suggest that the gunshot had travelled from the back of the leg to the front. Mr A was then referred to the hospital's orthopaedics department at 20:15, where Dr M, an orthopaedic surgeon, made a hand-drawn diagram of the left lower leg. The hand-drawn diagram, however, showed a gunshot wound travelling from front to back.

Mr A was alive and well, and he was referred to me to determine whether he had been shot from back to front or from front to back, because that would have far-reaching medico-legal consequences for the police, regarding the concept of reasonable force. Mr A himself couldn't even tell me if he had been shot from back to front or front to back, because the incident had happened so quickly.

The doctor's notes provided very limited data regarding the original wounds. How exactly they decided which was the entrance gunshot wound and which was the exit still remains a mystery to me. To make matters even more complicated, looking at the two circular scars on Mr A's left lower leg months later, I found it impossible even to determine if the original wounds were gunshot wounds at all. Healing and surgically modified wounds sadly complicate matters.

So how did I manage to solve this case? I requested the original

X-ray plates of the left lower leg from the hospital's admission section. Forensic pathologists and forensic radiologists use X-rays in evaluating gunshot wounds because they may reveal information about the angle and direction of fire. Small metallic fragments produced when a projectile strikes bone may lead directly to the projectile and clearly indicate the projectile's path. When a projectile strikes bone, its path can be deflected and fragmentation can occur, producing bone fragments that can act as additional small projectiles, thus increasing tissue damage. Furthermore, as a projectile travels through the body, it pushes tissue away from its path.

Based on the available X-ray data and Locard's Exchange Principle, I concluded that Mr A had been shot from front to back. To cut a long story short, Dr M from the Department of Orthopaedics was correct.

CASE STUDY 2

My profession has taught me to appreciate the rare and also to look at everyday objects in a different light. Unusual objects have been used as weapons: over the years I have seen people killed with ashtrays, horseshoes, dropper poles, pens, pencils and even toilet paper. In prisons, for example, toilet paper is tightly woven to create a noose. After ligature strangulation, the noose is simply flushed down the toilet.

I have seen people killed with a rolled-up magazine: the magazine is rolled up so tightly, it creates a baton-type weapon. I have seen people stabbed to death with a cigarette butt: in prisons, typically, the filter of a cigarette is melted with heat to create plastic which is then fashioned into a pointed and sharp-edged weapon such as a knife.

On a personal note, I am secretly terrified of paper shredders and all rotating machines, such as automatic car washes, which can accidentally catch a tie or a scarf or clothing and strangle and mangle the unwary.

12

Why this, why now?

I worked on the Marikana massacre, and while I will not go into the politics behind the tragedy, I want to discuss Locard's Exchange Principle in relation to this and other mass disasters.

On 16 August 2012, 34 miners, who were protesting about employment and salary-related matters at the Lonmin platinum mine between Rustenburg and Brits in the North West province of South Africa, were shot dead by police during a confrontation. Several other people also had gunshot injuries. This incident would become known as the Marikana Massacre.

Following the open-fire assault, 250 miners were arrested. On 22 August 2012, 20 autopsy examinations were conducted. On 23 August 2012, the remaining 14 autopsies were conducted. Five state doctors were engaged, of whom I was one. Ballistic experts, photographers and other assistants were also present, so as to assist with dry-hands specimen collection and C-arm (mobile X-ray) examination. Two independent forensic pathologists were also present.

As mentioned, it is outside of the remit of this book to discuss the politics of the tragedy and the events leading up to and surrounding the deaths, neither will I focus on my findings, nor on the key findings and recommendations of the Marikana Commission of Inquiry. Rather, I want to tell you how my experience highlighted challenges in the management of disasters from a forensic pathology aspect, and the insights that I gained. Most importantly, I wish to discuss Locard's Exchange Principle and mass disasters.

When my superiors phoned to inform me that I would be working on the Marikana case, I was on my way to work, having had only a spoonful of yoghurt and some coffee for breakfast that morning. What I didn't know then was that this small meal would have to keep me going for the entire day, because after that there was no time even to drink a cup of coffee.

As I have come to expect from working on cases of mass disasters, the working conditions were not ideal either. We felt pressurised and worked under very difficult conditions. We faced multiple challenges and they were tough autopsies to perform: the deceased were miners who had been big men, with muscular arms and large torsos from a lifetime of drilling into hard rock, and so the process took much discipline, willpower, stamina, mental fortitude and resilience.

By day two of the autopsies, I was already fatigued. My feet felt as if they were slushing around in my boots from my own sweat. There were also rumours that a certain politician was outside the mortuary while we were working. I was so very excited to meet the politician that I felt an electric thrill pass through my body. For the record, I am not a fan of any politician, either local or international, so the only way I can explain my excitement is that it must have been due to the extreme fatigue I felt.

All bodies had to be X-rayed one by one on a single C-arm. The X-ray service was ineffective, hazardous and inaccessible. There was also limited protection in accordance with the legal framework for radiation control in South Africa.[1] I personally received about one and a half hours of C-arm exposure during those three days because the personal protective equipment against X-rays was not up to standard according to the Hazardous Substances Act, Act 15 of 1973. At one point, I could literally feel my hands tingling while removing projectiles from the bodies. (I don't even want to mention exposure to other parts of my body, such as my thyroid gland.)

There was haste in the conducting of the autopsy examinations, which created perceived pressure. Usually, I like to take my time when doing autopsies: I like to settle down and perhaps even dawdle. I tend to take my autopsies step by step.

The medico-legal laboratory where the autopsies were performed was undergoing rehabilitation at the time, and there was poor infrastructure for the management of such an incident: the lighting was inadequate, there was limited air-conditioning and the space was a problem, with many interested parties concentrated in a very small area. There were also very few weighing scales and no insecticides, and pests were a problem (the chief pest being, of course, the fly). Also, the bodies were in a state of early decomposition.

The principle of Universal Precautions was practised, predicated on the assumption that all the autopsies carried a significant risk of transmitting disease, either by aerosols or through the use of sharp instruments. To prevent exposure, everyone wore surgical scrubs, boots, masks, head protection, aprons, sleeve covers and cut-resistant latex (or rubber) gloves.

Meticulous autopsies were conducted following the original version of the 1991 Minnesota Protocol, a set of international guidelines for the investigation of suspicious deaths, particularly those in which the responsibility of a state is suspected. Photographs were taken by forensic and police personnel. Clothing was removed layer by layer, with each item meticulously documented and carefully photographed. All bodies received full mobile C-arm fluoroscopy.

Each and every projectile was removed individually, documented, photographed and submitted with full appreciation of the chain of custody. Blood was taken for post-mortem ethanol concentration. Buccal swabs were also taken for DNA purposes. Full toxicology was performed in every case, which involved samples from peripheral blood, bile, stomach contents, liver, kidneys, urine and vitreous fluid. Since these were mine workers, cardiothoracic organs were also harvested according to the Occupational Diseases in Mines and Works Act, Act 78 of 1973, and sent to the National Institute for Occupational Health.

What saved us all were the basic principles of Locard's

Exchange Principle. Amidst the chaos and the poor conditions, it was Locard's teachings that guided the way: we documented, we collected and we preserved the evidence; simple as that, no more and no less.

For all our hard work, we were given a curt thank you and the authorities purchased us soft drinks, chicken, some cheese sauce and a few soggy chips after three days of intense autopsies under extreme conditions. The commission of inquiry that would follow cost a small fortune.

What I've learned is that mass disasters like the Marikana mining massacre tend to hit on the quiet days, when no one expects them. A 'mass disaster' may be defined as an occurrence with morbidity and/or mortality overstretching or overwhelming the local emergency services. It may be defined as natural, accidental or human-made.

Whether demonstrating against illegal wars, globalisation or new laws that infringe civil rights, large groups of people often gather to exercise their right to protest. It is part of the democratic way. However, sometimes things go wrong and either the police antagonise the protesters and violence breaks out, or there are troublemakers in the crowd that force the police to act to maintain law and order, using a reasonable amount of force.

Considering the potential for violent anarchy, hostile crowds and hordes of people, one question has repeatedly come to mind: how do you responsibly subdue a swathe of angry humans?[2]

This question again came to mind in July 2021, when violent unrest and looting that erupted in KwaZulu-Natal and Gauteng devastated businesses, hospitals and health services and also brought Covid-19 vaccinations to a halt. Lives were endangered by violence as well as by lack of access to medicine, medical treatment, oxygen, food and essential supplies. Some pharmacies were lost to looting and ambulances were attacked. Several services were suspended. There was large-scale destruction and damage to properties, and both the public and the private sector were hard-hit. There were also many protest-related injuries and deaths.

By late Wednesday, 14 July 2021, the high levels of unrest had begun to subside in some areas, after the South African National Defence Force (SANDF) fanned out across KwaZulu-Natal and parts of Gauteng, and law-abiding citizens worked with public and private security forces to guard areas.

What options exist for ensuring crowd control and preventing further violence? This is where the concept of less-than-lethal weaponry comes in – and who better than a friendly forensic pathologist to help contribute to this discussion?

Different terms exist in the literature for this phenomenon: less-lethal weapons, non-lethal weapons or sublethal weapons. In its most basic form, such a weapon is 'a discriminate weapon that is explicitly designed and used to incapacitate personnel or material while minimizing fatalities and undesired damage to property and environment'.[3] There are many ways of controlling riots: the traditional methods are water cannons, stun grenades and tear gas. Mechanical mechanisms have been used such as mobile (barbed wire) fencing and noise devices.

Certain pepper sprays have marker dyes in them which will mark the person who has been sprayed, for Locardian purposes. So too, with ATM bombings, there are dyes which will stain the culprits. Less-lethal weaponry includes a wide range of weapons based on the delivery of kinetic energy, incapacitating chemicals, including water cannons and electromagnetic energy devices. Some of these weapons can potentially cause serious injury or even death.

I specifically want to discuss the most responsible management of violent mobs and angry protestors with Locard's Exchange Principle in mind. What is the best possible way to control an angry mob?

In *Mostly Murder*, Sir Sydney Smith describes the situation at Abdin Palace in Egypt in the early part of the 1900s when he ran into a mob and thought the situation was critical. 'At that moment two mounted troopers of the Australian force came into the square. Their rifles remained in their holsters, and they were armed apparently with nothing but long canes and their distinctive slouch hats. As they approached in a nonchalant way, skilfully using their canes with encouraging cries such as '*Imshi!*' the raging crowd of thousands started to wilt away like snow in sunshine.'

According to Smith, this incident was a very good example of practical psychology.[4]

Rubber bullets are impact munitions made of rubber or other elastic materials that use kinetic energy, and they are among the oldest less-lethal weapon technologies. The shape and material of the bullets have been continuously modified since their first use in 1970.

Rubber bullets cause great pain and incapacitate the target. The majority of injuries are non-penetrating, although severe and fatal cases due to penetrating injuries or internal organ injuries have been reported. Rubber bullets and their injuries are familiar to few forensic pathologists because of the rarity of fatal incidents. I have, unfortunately, performed a number of autopsies on people who died due to rubber bullets. Mostly, these projectiles were fired at too close a range and penetrated the body of the victim, which resulted in death.

The typical rubber bullet measures 40 mm in diameter and weighs 30 grams. The elderly and the young are most at risk, although sometimes the healthy are injured and killed as well. The 40 mm rubber bullet may cause pulmonary contusion or contusions of the heart, liver or spleen, and chest impact may cause *commotio cordis* (a phenomenon in which a sudden blunt impact to the chest causes sudden death in the absence of cardiac damage). The rubber bullet may cause lacerations and contusions. The slightly rough surface of the sponge foam can cause strong skin traction, resulting in lacerations if it strikes the skin at an acute angle.[5] Suicide by rubber bullet has also been reported in the literature.[6]

Risk factors for death due to rubber bullets include short range of fire, young age, area of impact and bullet size, shape, mass and velocity on impact. The conditions of the target may also influence the severity of the results of trauma; for example, whether the target is wearing protective clothing, has thick hair, is fat or thin, is old or fragile, or is young or healthy. In other words, all the wounding factors have to do with the second part of Locard's Exchange Principle, namely the intensity, duration and nature of the contact.

Pepper spray was originally used for defence against bears, mountain lions, wolves and other dangerous predators, and is often referred to colloquially as bear spray.

Oleoresin capsaicin (OC) is an oily extract from hot pepper plants. OC extract is mostly composed of capsaicin, the same compound that gives spicy food its hotness. OC is the substance most likely to be found now in tear gas and pepper sprays. OC spray is a lachrymatory (causing tears) agent used in policing, riot control, crowd control and self-defence, including defence against dogs and bears. Its inflammatory effects cause the eyes to close, making it difficult to see. This temporary blindness allows officers to more easily restrain subjects and permits people in danger to use pepper spray in self-defence for an opportunity to escape. It also causes temporary discomfort and burning of the lungs, which results in shortness of breath.

Again, all the wounding factors have to do with the second part of Locard's Exchange Principle, namely the intensity, duration and nature of the contact.

Can exposure to this noxious irritant, capsaicin, cause or contribute to unexpected deaths? The answer is yes. Two cases of deaths have been described in relation to the use of OC spray.[7] Exposure to OC 'is basically as if your head is on fire, and you inhaled a hive of angry wasps', in the words of someone who was sprayed in the face with pepper spray.[8]

Pepper balls are like paint balls, except that instead of paint, they contain fine-powdered OC, or other chemical irritants. Upon impact, pepper balls burst and release their contents in a large dust cloud. So what should you do if you're exposed to tear gas or pepper spray? Get away from the area, and wash with copious amounts of soap and water, especially your hands and face.

Malodorants can also be used to incapacitate. Recently, the Israeli Defence Force came up with **Skunk**, a malodorant, non-lethal weapon used for crowd control. It is being marketed to militaries and law enforcement agencies around the world. The liquid's strong odour has been advertised as an improvement over other crowd control weapons such as rubber bullets and tear gas. Skunk is typically used when demonstrators become violent or engage in vandalism. There are specific rules of engagement for its use. It is said to contain an organic and non-toxic blend of baking powder, yeast and other ingredients.[9]

A BBC reporter described its effects as follows: 'Imagine the worst, most foul thing you have ever smelled. An overpowering mix of rotting meat, old socks that haven't been washed for weeks – topped off with the pungent waft of an open sewer. Imagine being covered in the stuff as it is liberally sprayed from a water cannon. Then imagine not being able to get rid of the stench for at least three days, no matter how often you try to scrub yourself clean.'[10]

It is reported that the smell is so potent it can linger on your clothes for months, if not years. The company that produces Skunk also sells a special soap, available to authorities but not the general public, that neutralises the smell of skunk water if officers are accidentally sprayed.[11] Skunk was criticised in a joint 2016 Physicians for Human Rights and International Network of Civil Liberties Organizations report on crowd control weapons published by the American Civil Liberties Union.[12]

The **Taser** was invented by Jack Cover in 1974 and marketed by Taser International, sixty years after a similar weapon had been written about in a young adult novel by Victor Appleton called *Tom Swift and His Electric Rifle* or *Daring Adventures in Elephant Land.* ('Taser' is Cover's tribute to the book – an acronym of 'Thomas A Swift's electric rifle'.) It is a handheld conducted electrical weapon (CEW), powered by two three-volt batteries, that induces neuromuscular incapacitation and pain by the application of a small electrical current.

The Taser fires two small dart-like electrodes, which stay connected to the main unit by conductive wire as they are propelled by small compressed-nitrogen charges. The physiological effect of CEWs is dependent on the distance between the two darts and their location on the body, in other words, it is a function of their 'spread'. At autopsy it is therefore critical to measure the distance between the two dart locations on the body. Tasers interrupt the ability of the brain to control the muscles in the body.

The electrical current stimulates both afferent sensory neurons, causing pain, and efferent motor neurons, causing involuntary skeletal muscle contraction. Non-lethal or low-lethality devices, like Tasers, typically have the objective of temporarily disabling the target person. The weapon is used to obtain physical and psychological control of violently re-sistive subjects.

There has been controversy in the press about the use of these weapons, and it has been claimed that they have been responsible for over three hundred deaths. Amnesty Inter-national believes strict limits should be placed on their use. While the report found there was 'no conclusive medical evidence' to indicate high risk of serious injury or death from the direct or indirect effects of CEW exposure in healthy, normal, non-stressed adults, it noted that the safety mar-gins may not be applicable in the case of small children, those with diseased hearts, the elderly, the pregnant and other potentially at-risk individuals.

When such less-lethal weaponry causes major injuries or death, the user and the manufacturer of the weapon may be criticised, and legal action can be brought against them. Taser International has defended the safety of its stun guns by spending millions on studies and forging close ties with police, medical examiners and consultants. When someone dies after an altercation involving one of these weapons, the manufacturer is quick to offer guidance to investigators.

Regarding exposure to CEWs, including Tasers, the sec-ond part of Locard's Exchange Principle once again comes to the fore, namely the intensity, duration and nature of the contact.

What then, have I learned from the trenches? My thoughts on this are essentially that we should simply *start* using less-than-lethal weaponry, because an injured protestor is better than a dead protestor. Law enforcement needs to phase out live weapons for crowd control and start using less-than-lethal weapons. This should also ensure fewer legal actions against the police and the military.

Furthermore, mass disasters and crowd eruptions are becoming frequent events in modern society, and regular drills and simulation exercises are required to prepare for such eventualities. We need joint operations centres (war rooms) with maps, giant plasma screens and real-time communication services. It's crucial to identify safer ways to control angry crowds.

We should also invest in the training of medico-legal doctors and support staff throughout Africa, adequate transport facilities for the mass transportation of bodies, adequate infrastructure to perform autopsies and store many bodies, stationery, support staff, mobile disaster management teams, upfront funding for disaster management, standard operating procedures and logistic plans. We need modern victim identification services. And, certainly, we need proper catering, please!

13

Rare and unusual cases

A 34-year-old male was involved in a single-vehicle motor vehicle accident as the driver of the car, in March 2021. He allegedly struck a rock or a solid object in an urban area and the vehicle rolled multiple times. He was found inside the vehicle and declared dead at the scene at approximately 15:00. No attempt at resuscitation was documented to have taken place.

Examination showed a well-nourished adult male with a height of 160 cm and a body mass of 71 kg. There were multiple fracture deformities involving the skull, facial bones, maxilla and mandible. Internal examination revealed an extensive comminuted fracture (the bone was broken in several places) of the calvarium and base of the skull. The dura was lacerated and the brain pulpified (residual mass of the brain 960 g). The airways contained brain matter. A section of the lungs revealed brain matter exuding from the smaller airways, with the left and right lung weighing 360 g and 440 g respectively. Histological examination of lung tissue showed the presence of brain tissue within the lumen of the distal bronchioles. There was pulmonary aspiration of brain matter in the lung tissue. ('Aspiration' is a term that refers to the accidental breathing in of food or fluid into the lungs.) Aspiration of brain matter is an extremely rare phenomenon, with only one other case described in the literature. The histology slides confirmed brain matter lodged deep within the distal airways.[1]

In other words, in one of the rarest cases I have ever seen, the man had breathed in his own brain!

One can only surmise how this might have happened. The pulpified brain tissue leaked through the fractured base of the skull and entered the upper airways. The cardiorespiratory centre is located in the brainstem and the brainstem controls breathing. The brainstem must obviously still have been functional, yet the front of the brain was pulpified. The pulpified brain tissue entered the airways through the base-of-skull fracture. There must have been some terminal (agonal) respirations before death, which caused the brain tissue to be breathed into the lungs. Impossible as it may sound, the histology photographs demonstrated brain tissue lodged deep within the distal airways. No other explanation seems plausible to explain this astonishing finding.

Rare cases such as the one just described are few in forensic pathology. Sometimes the textbooks predict that one will encounter a certain rare condition or event once in 100 000 occurrences. It might happen like this: you wake up, go to work and expect the day's bread-and-butter forensic cases, and there it suddenly is: the one-in-100 000 rare case. It is always very unexpected and totally unannounced, lying right there in front of you on the autopsy table.

Another highly uncommon sighting at an autopsy was a fully grown tapeworm with its head still intact. It was over two metres long. This is the sort of thing a medical practitioner usually sees once in a lifetime, or once in several lifetimes – especially in regions where one does not typically expect to find tapeworms. (These days many people deworm themselves with anthelmintics.[2])

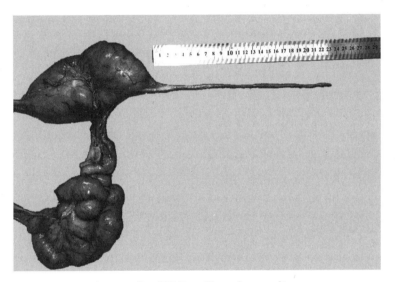

A appendix of 24,5cm. Normal appendixes measure between 8-10 cm in length.

That we as pathologists note facts such as these, no matter how arbitrary, adds to the cumulative knowledge of humankind. So, when I had a patient with an appendix 24.5 cm long, I could make a comparison with the largest appendix ever removed, as recorded by Guinness World Records: it measured 26 cm. It was removed from a 72-year-old patient, Safranco August from Croatia, during an autopsy at the Ljudevit Jurak University Department of Pathology, Zagreb, Croatia, in August 2006.

There are the very rare incidents which lead to death, such as the time I came across a fire extinguisher used in a suicide.[3] This unusual case helped elucidate a forensic dilemma which has been around since 1939.[4]

First some background. 'Pneumomediastinum, also known as mediastinal emphysema, is a condition in which air is present in the mediastinum (the space in the chest between the two lungs). This can be caused by a traumatic injury [such as drowning or lightning] or in association with pneumothorax or other diseases.'[5] At autopsy, pneumomediastinum looks like bubble wrap when one removes the sternal plate. It is not a pneumothorax (the presence of air or gas in the cavity between the lungs and the chest wall, causing collapse of the lung – a typically fatal condition). The lung does not collapse with pneumomediastinum and so it is not a fatal condition.

The question is: how does the air get into this area? In 1939 Macklin came up with a theory as to how air arrived in the mediastinum. This became known as the Macklin Effect. The Macklin Effect relates to a three-step pathophysiologic process, namely: blunt traumatic alveolar ruptures, air dissection along bronchovascular sheaths, and spreading of this pulmonary interstitial emphysema into the mediastinum.

Back to the suicide case. It provided strong evidence in support of the presence of the Macklin Effect. It also provided the first visual evidence of the phenomenon. On its last inspection, 13 days prior to the incident, the fire extinguisher had a working pressure of approximately 1 400 kPa (203 psi). In 2017, the deceased – who had a known psychiatric history, having been diagnosed with an underlying mood disorder – was found dead in the back garden of a private psychiatric hospital. The brick wall behind the deceased showed a shadow area created by the fine white powder. He was found lying on the ground, face up, covered with the powder, and an empty fire extinguisher was present to the left of his body. The label of the fire extinguisher showed it to contain a 34–40 per cent mono ammonium phosphate base.[6] Examination of the scene suggested that the deceased was sitting at the time the fire extinguisher discharged.

Autopsy examination showed an adult white male with fine white powder covering the entire face and also present within the mouth and sinuses and lining the upper airways. There was subcutaneous emphysema in the cheeks (this occurs when air gets into tissues under the skin) and congestion of the eyes. When the thoracic cavity was opened, approximately 500 g of the fine white powder was found within the right thoracic cavity. The oesophagus was ruptured and traumatic emphysema of the posterior sternum wall was present (pneumomediastinum). The ethmoid bones (square bones at the root of the nose) were fractured due to barotrauma.

The fire extinguisher powder did not play a significant role in the death of the individual. The air pressure that caused the powder to be distributed was critical here. These findings were appreciated upon observing the fractured ethmoid bones as well as the extensive laceration of the oesophagus. (There is scant literature on fire-extinguisher-related deaths.)

At histology, some of the alveoli were dilated, whereas others appeared ruptured. There was irregular distension of the alveoli at places. There was a foreign substance (with a crystal-like lattice) present within some of the distal alveoli. At places, the lung tissue had the appearance of emphysema. Upon polarisation, birefringent (when a ray of light splits into two) material was noted in a bronchovascular distribution and within the sub-pleural membranes.[7] The fire extinguisher contained amorphous silica – which is magic stuff to us forensic pathologists. Silica shines bright under a polarisation microscope. The distribution of the birefringent material provided the first real visual evidence in support of the Macklin Effect. Locard's Exchange Principle helped provide the means to visually demonstrate this very rare phenomenon.

Staying on the rare, unique and sometimes famous individuals have also turned up on my autopsy table, including a president. (Forensic pathologists play an important role in society. Who else will diagnose how a president died? The findings could plunge a country into war or create peace. Being a forensic pathologist is therefore a critical occupation.)

I was one of six pathologists who helped performed the autopsy on a deceased president. The standard of care was higher than anything I had seen in my life: the level of detail, the momentum and the resources. Presidential VIP protection was involved, and the case involved 'onion skin' policing for many of the suburbs surrounding the mortuary: a drone hovered silently above the mortuary, and there were laser beams around the fridge in which the dead president's body was stored. Post-mortem cosmetic experts embalmed and preserved the body. (With the late president, the post-mortem cosmetic expert was so proficient that few would have even realised that an autopsy had been performed at all.)[8]

At times, forensic pathologists are asked to review a body, especially one which has been exhumed or which has been under the care of a post-mortem cosmetic expert, and Locard's Exchange Principle comes into play once again. What were the original injuries that caused the death, and what were the artefactual changes caused by post-mortem cosmetic expert?

According to the cosmetic expert, of whom there are only a handful in South Africa, the body of the president would be preserved for up to 40 years.

CASE STUDY 1

According to the available history, when the car of the 29-year-old male concerned overturned and hit a wall, he died due to a head injury. At autopsy diffuse brain injury was present and we noticed that a small piece of glass had penetrated the left occipital bone of the skull.

What was remarkable was that this wound mimicked a projectile injury. A small shard of glass had penetrated the left occipital aspect of the skull and this bony wound defect was located approxi

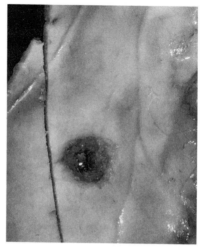

*A small piece of glass had penetrated the left occipital bone of the skull.
To the uninformed, this looked exactly like a glass projectile
penetrating the skull bone.*

mately 6 cm posterior and lateral from the greater wing of the left sphenoid bone. The wound defect also showed inward bevelling of bone. The tabula externa defect measured approximately 1 cm in diameter and the tabula interna defect measured approximately 1.5 cm in diameter.

To the uninitiated, it would have looked as if he had been shot with a glass bullet.

CASE STUDY 2

I once performed an autopsy on a deceased pedestrian who had been wearing 23 layers of clothing. It took us longer to undress him than to perform the autopsy.

156

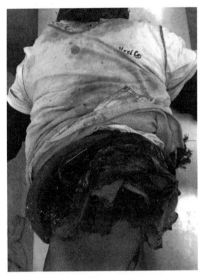

We had to remove 23 layers of clothing to perform the autopsy on this man. Each item of clothing had to be carefully removed, every pocket checked and each clothing label noted.

A book could be written on the pathology of clothing. Apart from the incriminating traces of materials that may be found on clothing, it can reveal a mass of information about the identity, habits and actions of their wearer.[9] Your clothing, your shoes, your belt, your jewellery – all contain different clues.

Clothing is a form of self-expression and can reveal much about a person. Nowadays clothing hardly has any protective value and is more often about fashion. Clothing can tell us forensic pathologists what work the deceased did, especially if they are wearing a uniform.

By investigating their clothing, forensic scientists have even helped to catch ATM bombers. When an ATM machine explodes, 'bomb dust' settles in the lower seams of their trousers, or turn-ups. Evidence from the ATM bombing can therefore be found in their turn-ups.

Why the deceased pedestrian who arrived on my autopsy table was wearing 23 layers of clothing will forever remain a mystery to me. Was he a psychiatric patient? Was he very cold? Or was he simply a hoarder of clothing?

CASE STUDY 3

There is currently a global opioid crisis. So how does one adjudicate a drug overdose death? How do you make a fair and accurate assessment of these cases within a short timeframe and are they suicide, accident or misadventure? These cases are understandably also often highly sensitive and emotive.

In 2020, two months after the start of the Covid-19 lockdown, an elderly couple were found dead in their apartment. A typed and signed suicide 'death pact' was found at the scene and no foul play was suspected by the police. The couple had apparently planned to end their lives with dignity through assisted suicide at a clinic in Switzerland. However, when the Covid-19 pandemic broke out and countries went into lockdown in March 2020, their plans were upended.

Their deaths occurred in May 2020. According to their son, it was a premeditated pact that had been carefully planned, as his parents had stockpiled fentanyl patches which his mother had used for non-specific neck pain management. The father had a background in chemistry, mathematics and physics.

Since this was deemed an unnatural death, a medico-legal autopsy was arranged and was performed by me the following day. The 76-year-old woman had 15 fentanyl 75 μg/h (12.6 mg) transdermal patches neatly secured with adhesive plasters to the upper anterior chest region. The 79-year-old man had ten fentanyl 75 μg/h (12.6 mg) transdermal patches neatly adhering to the anterior thorax and left cubital fossa region. No other fatal external injuries to the bodies could be identified. Internal organ findings were non-specific. Signed end-of-life directives were also found.

Suicide pacts are very rare, with pacts between two or more people making up approximately only 0.6–2.5 per cent of all suicides. Most suicide pacts occur between married couples or those in a relationship or friendship, or where both have a history of mental disorder or chronic medical illness. Suicide pacts have also been arranged via the internet and between like-minded individuals.

Fentanyl is a strong analgesic with a potency approximately a hundred times stronger than that of morphine. First brought to the market in the late 1950s, it is currently available in a range of different products. Today, the patches are mainly used in the long-term management of chronic pain or for cancer patients. People have come up with many ingenious ways of getting access to fentanyl, which is basically an opioid related to morphine.

Fentanyl addicts have been known to ingest whole patches, masticating them like chewing gum, injecting them or heating up the patches on a square of foil and inhaling the smoke through a tube. Another common method is the so-called and self-explanatory 'tea bag': users literally soak the patches in water like tea bags. Rectal insertion has also been described.

The easiest method is to apply multiple transdermal patches at once, as in this case.[10] The fentanyl reaches the bloodstream through the transdermal devices. The intensity, the duration and the nature of the materials determines the extent of the transfer. This case demonstrates Locard's Exchange Principle in a variety of ways.

CASE STUDY 4

In November 2022, I performed the autopsy on an adult man who had sustained multiple gunshot wounds to the body. There were perforating gunshot wounds through the limbs, the chest and the abdomen, and an atypical gunshot wound on the lateral aspect of the left thigh.

The wound on the left thigh measured two centimetres in diameter and the edges were irregular. Within the central aspect of this wound we discovered a malformed R2 coin. It transpired that the R2 coin was in the deceased's left trouser pocket when it was hit by the incoming projectile. It is particularly rare for a projectile to strike a coin in a person's pocket and for both coin and projectile to penetrate the body,.

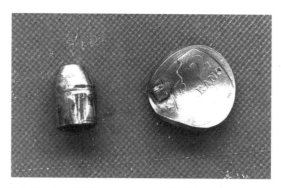

The R2 coin (right) and the projectile (left) that hit it as it passed through the victim's pocket.

CASE STUDY 5

One day when I was post-call, I greeted a colleague as I walked down the corridors of our pathology building. I noticed what I thought were electric iron burn marks on his white long-sleeved shirt. On seeing this, I remarked that he should perhaps purchase himself a steam iron or watch YouTube videos on 'How to Iron'. I was reminded of an unusual and tragic case where a victim tried to commit suicide by electrocuting themselves with an electric iron in the bathtub. I mentioned to him that the iron marks on his white shirt looked very similar to the iron imprint burn marks on the skin of the victim. To my absolute embarrassment, my colleague informed me that he was actually wearing a designer white shirt with a subtle brown fern-like pattern on the material. At this point I realised that perhaps I needed to get some rest and take some leave.

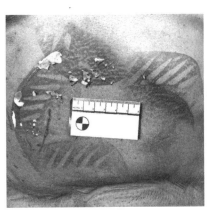 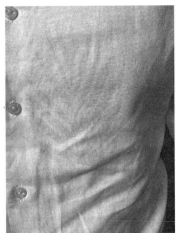

Left: *The appearance of burn marks from an electric iron on the skin.*

Right: *What I had thought was a burn mark from an electric iron turned out to be a fern pattern on an expensive designer shirt*

14

Occupational health and safety

By now, you already know that the mortuary can be a very dangerous place. There are risks such as slippery floors, sharp corners, knives and saws, and points of super-sharp needles. There are also biological hazards, such as hepatitis, HIV and other blood-borne diseases. The many potential hazards present within a body are generally unknown at the start of the autopsy. So it will come as no surprise that many pathologists have tragically died or become ill while performing their normal duties.

I've read about a pathologist who died of streptococcal infection after sustaining minor cutaneous injury during autopsy on person with the same disease;[1] there are at least two records of pathologists who acquired hepatitis;[2] glanders was fatally transmitted to a veterinary prosector who had a drop of infected horse blood enter his mouth;[3] two cases of Creutzfeldt-Jakob disease have been documented in histology technicians working in separate neuropathology labs;[4] and prosectors have died of autopsy-transmitted Marburg, Ebola and Lassa haemorrhagic fevers. Some theories suggest spread by direct cutaneous inoculation.

Many people have asked me what the difference in risk level is between a forensic pathologist and a surgeon. From an infection point of view, the surgeon chiefly has to protect the patient from the surgeon, which is why surgeons work in sterile environments. Surgeons are often exposed to extreme risks. Forensic pathologists have to protect themselves from the patients. We do not work in sterile environments. Forensic pathologists are often exposed to extreme extreme risks. In the autopsy room, we as forensic pathologists are always in danger: we have to protect ourselves from the patients.

Our patients may have died due to extreme exposure to trauma, infection or chemicals. Forensic pathologists are often exposed to the same infections, chemicals, risks and hazards. In murder cases, the forensic pathologist may also risk exposure to the killers, be they gang members or the mafia.

That is why the title of this book is *Risking Life for Death*. More often than not, forensic pathologists place their life at risk for another's death.

For this reason, I want to write a bit about occupational health and safety at autopsy, which of course also obey Locard's Exchange Principle. This chapter will highlight the consequences of dangerous contacts. There may be dangerous foreign bodies hidden within the corpse, or hidden sharp objects may be located within the body or the clothing. I once had a fully cocked and loaded handgun fall out of a pocket. There was also an occasion when a screwdriver (used as a weapon) had been hidden inside a sock. Razor-sharp needles and needle fragments inside pockets of intravenous drug users have sometimes pricked unsuspecting forensic personnel. So, pockets must always be patted – never simply stick your hand into one.

I have discovered some other crazy stuff in pockets over the years. (Used condoms and tissues stained with coughed tuberculosis blood come to mind.) Best practice is to first X-ray or CT scan a body.

Ideally, all bodies need pre-autopsy screening; however, this is a luxury. Most often we get 'street cases' – bodies straight off the streets, which could be from anywhere in the world (given that the world is currently suffering a migrant crisis and that borders are generally porous). Refugees often enter a country with their endemic diseases.

Biologic agents can cause infection and death. We classify these from high-risk to low-risk.

- Category A: (high-level risk) such as smallpox, anthrax, Ebola and Marburg viruses.
- Category B: such as Q fever, glanders, ricin toxin, and vibrio cholera.
- Category C: such as tick-borne haemorrhagic fever and multidrug-resistant TB.

From a health and safety perspective at autopsy in South Africa, the most dangerous biologic agents (from a day-to-day service-delivery point of view) are: mycobacterium tuberculosis, human immunodeficiency virus, hepatitis B and C, and miscellaneous infections such as Neisseria meningitides.

One of the most dangerous bodies to perform an autopsy on is a prion case. Prions are abnormal, pathogenic agents that are transmissible and are able to induce abnormal folding of specific normal cellular proteins, called prion proteins, that are found most abundantly in the brain. Prions cause transmissible spongiform encephalopathies, like mad cow disease. Preferably, we do not want to perform an autopsy on any prion case. However, there are times when such an autopsy has to be performed, especially when there are medico-legal issues at stake. This is about as dangerous as it gets in forensic pathology.

Such an autopsy is limited to one experienced pathologist and minimal staff. The pathologist will require high-quality personal protective equipment, disposable, waterproof gowns, cut-resistant gloves and powered air-purifying respirators. The autopsy table should be covered with super-absorbent sheets and waterproof backing – which require incineration afterwards. The brain is carefully removed and placed in a plastic bag and weighed, and immediately placed in 10% neutral buffered formalin.

It is almost impossible to inactivate prions. They are characterised by extreme resistance. Irradiation, boiling, dry heat, formalin and alcohol are all useless. Textbooks suggest high concentrations of sodium hydroxide, which is a caustic base, and alkali that decomposes proteins at ordinary ambient temperatures. Prions can be inactivated by steam sterilisation, which is accomplished in an autoclave. There are four parameters to steam sterilisation: steam, pressure, temperature and time. Autoclaving at 132°C for four and a half hours has been shown to inactivate prions. Statistically, if one looks at the number of autopsies performed in South Africa, it is most likely that some forensic pathologists have already been exposed to prion disease without their knowledge or awareness.

Then there are chemical risks. Sometimes one gets a contaminated body. The body may be covered with any type of chemical contaminant. The outer body may be covered in organophosphates or even nerve gas (tabun, sarin, soman, GF, VX). There may be radioactive contaminants on or within the body, either deliberately or due to treatment.

Humans have a long history with chemical agents used in war. Many of these chemical agents are still circulating in societies. Forensic pathologists may be exposed to blood agents (such as hydrogen cyanide or cyanogen chloride), blister agents (such as lewisite, sulphur mustards or phosgene oxime) or even heavy metals, (such as arsenic, lead or mercury). There may be cyanide within the stomach (which can overcome the pathologist upon examining the gastric contents).

There may be volatile toxins on the body (such as benzene or chloroform). The deceased may have died due to pulmonary agents (such as phosgene or chlorine) or incapacitating agents (such as any of the pesticides).[5]

The deceased may have died due to explosives, and may be covered with traces of ammonium nitrate or fuel oil, or flammable gases such as gasoline or propane. There may even be poisonous industrial gases involved (such as the cyanides or nitriles). The toughest autopsies are when the deceased has been exposed to corrosive industrial acids and bases (such as nitric acid or sulphuric acid).

Disposing of these chemicals is very important. You don't just pour them down the drain or flush them down a toilet. Locard's Exchange Principle must be remembered: the chemical will rear its ugly little head somewhere else in society. Disposal of dangerous chemicals requires specialised services with formal disposal protocols.

Then there are miscellaneous risks. Greenfield filters, metal devices implanted into the inferior vena cava, the body's largest vein, used for the prevention of pulmonary emboli, are super sharp and can cut straight through the gloves of an unwary forensic pathologist. Rarely, forensic pathologists have been shocked by implanted cardioverter defibrillators. And, of course, there is always the possibility of strange projectiles, such as the Winchester Black Talon bullet, known for its unique construction and sharp petal shape after expansion following impact, which can penetrate straight through a glove and injure forensic staff.[6]

The autopsy of a chemically, biologically or radioactively contaminated body requires decontamination. This process is a super-specialisation and requires removing and chemically degrading the clothing. In a mortuary setting we create three zones: the hot zone, the warm zone and the cold zone. The hot zone is the area contaminated by the agent. The warm zone is the area immediately surrounding the hot zone. The cold zone is the area outside the warm zone.

You never know when you are going to perform an autopsy on a hazardous or high-risk body. Hence, we always need to be prepared. We treat all bodies as potentially deadly, which is a key reason why better-prepared autopsy infrastructure and funding are always necessary. In my opinion, all mortuaries should function at biosafety level 3, *at least*. All medico-legal mortuaries require proper ventilation, with negative pressure. Biosafety level 4 cases should preferably be performed in a specialised or mobile unit. Hazardous cases should use no aerosol-generating procedures (in other words, no oscillating head saw, which is a power tool that causes more bone dust than a manual band saw). All staff should wear N-95 respirators and other excellent-quality personal protective devices.

All staff require regular biosafety training. In our mortuary we have the saying '1.5 keeps you alive' – because we try to stand at least 1.5 metres away from everyone at all times. This decreases the risk of a needle prick accident, a splash or worse. All staff should have their immunisation status checked for the most common diseases. There should be periodic screening for tuberculosis, either by a chest X-ray or by other means. All personnel should have immediate and easy access to health care after exposure.

Before starting in the field of forensics, every staff member should have a full medical check-up, physical and psychological. This is important for proving that you actually acquired your injury on duty, and didn't enter the occupation with it. All staff need to undergo a crash-course in occupational health and safety at autopsy. If you don't understand the risks, you will get injured or die. And everyone must understand safe sharps practice. ('Sharps' in this context is a medical term for devices with sharp points or edges that can puncture or cut the skin.)

Forensic personnel require excellent equipment. Occupational health and safety is a super-speciality these days, and obviously much more can be done to advance health and safety in our workplace. These are the minimum requirements.

CASE STUDY 1

Once I had to collected blood from a deceased pedestrian to test for ethanol and other drugs. For this, I used a post-mortem blood alcohol sampling kit. According to the protocol, we typically collect femoral blood or brachial vessel blood (far away from the stomach, because alcohol has been known to diffuse away from the stomach to nearby blood vessels and artificially raise the blood alcohol level).

For the collection of post-mortem blood, we use a 20 ml McCartney bottle made of glass, with a cap containing Teflon lining and an anti-leak mechanism that seals airtight, which is sterile. The McCartney bottle typically contains a preservative (sodium fluoride) and an anti-coagulant (potassium oxalate). These powdered substances keep the blood fluid and prevent post-mortem production of alcohol by bacteria.

Anyway, I had collected the blood and was busy closing the cap, when the whole bottle suddenly cracked and shattered in my hand. A glass shard cut through my glove and into my palm. I could feel the warm blood soak my hand! I had a three-centimetre incised wound on the palm of my right hand.

I immediately tested the patient for HIV and a host of other bio-logic agents. (The patient was HIV positive). I also washed, scrubbed and irrigated my wound. I reported this as an injury on duty, and I had to go on immediate full post-exposure prophylaxis (all the antiretroviral drugs) and for full debriefing and counselling. I would have to have protected sex for the next six months. Luckily, I never seroconverted.

Most of my colleagues in forensic pathology have had similar incidents. Colleagues have been stabbed by the sharp ends of rib bones, the frontal crest of the frontal bone of the skull, and even the styloid process. Incidentally, HIV infection is higher in forensic autopsy populations than in the general public (because of over-representation of intravenous drug users among decedents at autopsy). The transmission risk with infected blood for HIV is 0.3% per exposure.[7] However, the overall risk of seroconversion after contact with HIV positive blood is relatively low.

There is only one well-documented case of HIV transmission at autopsy, in which a scalpel blade injury to the hand led to seroconversion of a consultant pathologist.[8] The risk of seroconversion after occupational exposure depends on the viral load in the patient, the volume of fluid inoculated and the susceptibility of the health care worker, including whether or not they receive post exposure prophylaxis. Other factors include the depth of injury, terminal illness in the source patient, and procedures involving the direct placement of needles into blood vessels.[9]

In other words, here again the second part of Locard's Exchange Principle applies, namely intensity, duration and nature of contact.

15

How to be a medical detective in your own life

In May 2021 I fell off my mountain bike and fractured my left wrist. It was during the KAP sani2c, a three-day, 265-kilometre mountain bike race, which takes place in KwaZulu-Natal. The event begins on a small sheep farm near the Sani Pass in the southern Drakensberg and continues through the Midlands, mist belts, dairy and timber farms and indigenous forests, and down a breathtaking pass into the Umkomaas Valley, before criss-crossing a nature reserve and sugar cane farms that eventually deliver mountain bikers onto the shores of the Indian Ocean.

On Day 2, during the Umkomaas Valley descent, known as the Umko Drop, I fell off my mountain bike and sustained a fracture to my left wrist. It was something the orthopaedic surgeons would call a 'die-punch' fracture – essentially, a very bad fracture involving multiple bones of my wrist. Due to the nature of the terrain, it was very difficult to get help on the mountain and somehow I had to get to the first water point (some 30 km from where I had the accident), or some place where I could get medical assistance.

What followed was three hours of hell: I strapped my wrist with duct tape and sticks. And after three excruciating hours, I managed to get help, and an ambulance then drove me 82 km to the nearest hospital, where I was treated. The fracture was reduced by the ER doctor and I was placed in a plaster of Paris cast. However, the fracture required formal reduction and internal fixation with plate and screws, so I was referred for formal orthopaedic surgery.

After Covid-19 nasal swabs had been declared negative, I was booked and declared fit for orthopaedic surgery. I arrived in the ward, where there were three other patients: a gunshot robbery victim, a robbery victim who had jumped out of a two-storey building and fractured his ankle, and another poor victim of crime. I was the only non-crime-related patient in the ward, and the mood among the orthopaedic patients was sombre.

On my bed were the disposable theatre clothes that I would have to don before surgery. I put them on in the bathroom and walked quietly and solemnly to my bed. Little did I know that I had accidentally placed the theatre gown on the wrong way around, and as for the underpants, well, I had placed those on my head. (In my defence: I thought it was a surgical scrub cap, because in forensic pathology we typically wear disposable surgical scrub caps. In retrospect, I was quite amused by the fancy two holes for my ears . . .)

As I walked into the ward, a formidable sister approached me, and in front of all the other patients, all she could say was: 'Professor . . .' before they all burst into fits of laughter.

Being sick and in pain often doesn't allow for clear and crisp thinking (as my little demonstration in the hospital, preparing for surgery, indicates). And yet, most people only start questioning their own health when they are sick. Why not rather question your own health while you are feeling brilliant? When you wake up feeling great, that is precisely the right time to start interrogating your life: what did you eat and drink the previous day? What did you do the previous day or week for you to be feeling so incredible? You can only think clearly about disease and pathology when your mind is sharp and healthy. Imagine flicking a crystal wine glass that resonates in clear harmony for minutes, versus flicking a plastic bucket! This is the difference between a clear mind versus a foggy one. Therefore let us discuss disease, pestilence and death right now, while you are (hopefully) healthy and in good spirits.

You wake up and you are feeling tired: maybe you didn't sleep well, maybe you feel a bit weak, or just not on point. Hopefully, you have enough insight into yourself to know when you are not functioning at factory settings. Thinking like a medical detective is a valuable approach to everyday situations – especially in a world where we are being constantly bombarded with information. Look at all the miracle cures, wonder diets, ideologies, conspiracy theories, urban myths, and certain medical and psychiatric claims. All of these are accompanied by what's referred to as 'evidence'. How often do we critically interrogate this evidence? What you eat and what you drink – your fuel – play an important part in the functioning of the machine that is your body.

The health of the nation astounds me at autopsy. I often see fatty streaks deposited on the intimal surfaces of the large blood vessels in young people who are just 20 to 30 years old. Sometimes I notice an average anterior abdominal fat-wall thickness for young adults of about three to four centimetres. (The normal anterior abdominal fat-wall thickness is approximately one to two centimetres.) Some people seem to be suffering from chronic carbohydrate poisoning. Out of all the slow poisonings, I think the chronic intake of bad carbohydrates is probably the most insidious.

Most people are oblivious to cause and effect. Take migraines, for example: there is no reason to get a migraine. Mammals are not meant to get migraines, so surely these must be a reaction to something?

Forensic pathologists are medical detectives in white coats, and we have to dig until we find a root cause. Because of this, we learn to ask basic questions which go to the heart of the validity of any claim. If someone approaches me with a fantastic claim, I say: 'That's nice. Let's prove it.' Although the more correct scientific response would be: 'That's nice. Now let's disprove it.' The same should apply to how you approach your life and your health.

When dealing with health problems, you need to know that there are only eight aetiological[1] reasons why living creatures get sick or die:

1. An infection: a virus, bacteria, prion, parasite or some or another bug. SARS-CoV-2 is an example of a viral infection. There are only three outcomes to

an infection: you kill it, it kills you, or you become a carrier of it.

2. Cancer: the cancer may be benign or malignant. The origin of the neoplasm may be due to a multitude of factors – all of which obey Locard's Exchange Principle.

3. Mechanical: in other words, you were injured by a force. Forces may be kinetic or non-kinetic, which can cause wounding. Even pregnancy falls into this category: cephalopelvic disproportion is a mechanical matter, where the foetal head is too big to pass through the birth canal. Maybe you have disc degeneration, where the disk tissue mechanically impinges on one of your spinal cord nerves.

4. Reactive: you are reacting to something. Maybe your body does not like something and forms an attack against it. (Perhaps the bacteria your body is attacking look like your own body.) Rheumatic fever, for example, is a disease that can affect the heart, joints, brain and skin. Rheumatic fever can develop if strep throat, scarlet fever or strep skin infections are not treated properly. Bacteria called group A streptococcus (group A strep) cause these infections. Rheumatic carditis is associated with antistreptococcal antibodies. Your body thinks it is attacking the bacteria, whereas your body is actually attacking itself.

5. Iatrogenic (induced unintentionally by a physician or surgeon or by medical treatment or diagnostic procedures) illness is when your state of ill health

175

is caused by medical treatment. Maybe it is the result of a mistake made in treatment by a nurse, doctor or pharmacist.

6. Poisoning: too much of a substance has been taken. 'The dose makes the poison'[2] is an adage credited to Paracelsus. It is a basic principle of toxicology that a substance can produce harmful effects only if it reaches a susceptible biological system within the body in high enough concentrations. Even too much water can poison you.

7. Psychological: perhaps the sickness arose in your mind or is related to your mental or emotional state.

8. Congenital or genetic: you were born with it and perhaps the cause is in your genes.

All of these causes tend to adhere to Locard's Exchange Principle. You get sick or you die when you are exposed to one of the aforementioned eight causes. To be a medical detective you need to think in terms of cause and effect and interchange theory (contact theory). I am constantly on the lookout for these eight causes when it comes to sickness or death. You can apply the eight aetiological reasons to dead seals washing up on a beach, to dead crocodiles floating down a river, to the sudden, unexplained death of a human, or even to your hay fever.

To catch a murderer requires energy. A medico-legal investigation is time-, cost- and labour-intensive. As you have seen in this book, you need to devote yourself entirely to the one issue at hand. If you really want to determine the pure cause of something, you should not waste your time on lesser stuff. If you really want to become a medical detective, you must devote all your time and energy to solving that one specific problem. Therefore, determine which problems are solvable and which are probably not solvable. Devote your time, energy and resources only to the solvable problems; as you should for your life and your health.

In the beginning of this book, I mentioned that I have been concerned about the level of commitment and professionalism these days. The 'will to solve it' needs to be there. You need the right people with the right mind-set and the right attitude to solve problems. Put a good manager in a bad store, and you will have a good store. Put a bad manager in a good store, and you will have a bad store. With the right people, time, energy and resources, I believe all our earthly problems can be solved.

The thing that kills you is not necessarily the thing that you were worrying about. Your reality is not necessarily the true reality. Your reality is only a small percentage of the bigger picture. Daily exposure to news, social media, your friends, your work colleagues and your family creates your perceived way of viewing the world. Daily exposure to certain narratives and other people's interpretations of what is happening all around may well end up becoming your version. For example, if you are working in a cancer ward, you may think cancer is pervasive, whereas, in fact, only a small percentage of the population develop cancer. The world is much bigger and much more complex than any one person's perceived reality and private logic. Locard's Exchange Principle is again at play here: daily, people are being exposed to stuff and infected with stuff – sold stuff and proselytised. How many of your own ideas are actually your own? Did you decide to buy that item, or were you sold it by a salesperson? Your world is mainly the books, television series, podcasts and conversations which you have been exposed to. Please note that there is also a large chunk of information which you have not been exposed to. I can only diagnose what I have read, seen, heard and know. I only know what I have studied and so logically will not be able to diagnose what I do not know. *I don't know what I don't know.*

Proselytisation has a lot to do with Locard's Exchange Principle: you will see that books written on any subject are typically written by those who want to convert, or attempt to convert, a person from one religion, belief or opinion to another. So too with an idea that is trending: if you had not heard about it, seen it or read about it, you most likely would not have known about it. You would not know if you were left wing, right wing, communist, socialist, fascist or vegetarian. It is highly unlikely that you would have invented these ideologies all by yourself. You would not know anything about them. You have been proselytised through Locard's Exchange Principle. Stretched by a new idea, the mind never returns to its original dimensions.

The thing that kills you generally sideswipes from the left or the right or comes from behind – the explosion, the accidental fall, the car crash, the electrocution. All of these are the hidden risks in society. No amount of preparation can decrease your risks for certain conditions that can injure or kill you. You may try to engineer a safer society by designing safer roads, or you can try to learn from the mistakes and deaths of others. Sadly, humans are humans and we rarely learn from history. Even within the safest of societies, there will always be a need for a forensic pathologist.

To be a medical detective in your own life, whether it be to diagnose your own health, to make sense of everyday information or to solve any other problem, keep in mind the key points of Locard's Exchange Principle:_

1. Every contact leaves a trace. Trace evidence is typically left at or taken from the scene.
2. Look for the clues (traces), which tell the story.
3. Look for blatant signs and also subtle signs of transfer.
4. Almost everything leaves traces of itself.
5. Specific contacts leave specific traces.
6. Locard's Exchange Principle works on the subatomic level and the cosmic level.
7. You can discover the existence of something based on its interaction with other things.
8. Crime scenes can be recreated using Locard's Exchange Principle.
9. The extent of transfer depends on three variables, namely the intensity of contact, the duration of contact and the nature of the material.
10. Even tampering leaves a trace.

11. If you find no traces on the body, look towards the environment for traces.
12. Finally, understand cause and effect (causation).

16

A recap of
Locard's Exchange Principle

In my career, I have attended death scenes of people on the toilet, in their television rooms, on the soccer field, in the swimming pool, in their bedrooms and while travelling. When I drive around my city, I drive up some streets and realise that, at some point over the years, I was in that particular house for a murder scene, I was on that particular street corner for a rape-homicide, it was in that particular rubbish bin that I found the discarded products of conception, it was that particular apartment building which had a jumper from the eleventh floor.

I have seen people who have died while shopping for brand-new clothing, on their wedding night, at their bachelor parties, while fine-dining and even during intense lovemaking. I have seen people who have died when they were highly motivated and when they really seemed to be enjoying their lives. Surely, the worst time to die must be when you are living your best life?

There is something extraordinarily rare and precious about life. Yet, every day, from my perspective, people seem to be taking their own lives, or those of other people. Noticing this much death makes one acutely aware of the hidden risks and dangers of society. It also makes one aware of the 'contacts' you have in everyday life.

If I were to summarise Locard's Exchange Principle, I would say that it is pervasive throughout our lives. It is the grand unifying theory through which all things are connected. You can trace and track anything back to its source, via its 'contacts'. You can find the ultimate truth if you dig deep enough and follow the clues to their ultimate conclusion.

Recall that Dr Edmond Locard was a pioneer in forensic science who became known as the Sherlock Holmes of Lyon, France, and formulated the basic principle of forensic science: *'Every contact leaves a trace,'* or *'With contact between two items, there will be an exchange.'* Paul L Kirk[1] expressed Locard's Exchange Principle as follows:

> Wherever he steps, whatever he touches, whatever he leaves, even unconsciously, will serve as silent evidence against him. Not only his fingerprints or his footprints, but his hair, the fibers from his clothes, the glass he breaks, the tool mark he leaves, the paint he scratches, the blood or semen he deposits or collects – all these and more bear mute witness against him. This is evidence that does not forget. It is not confused by the excitement of the moment. It is not absent because human witnesses are. *It is factual evidence.* Physical evidence cannot be wrong; it cannot perjure itself; it cannot be wholly absent. Only its interpretation can err. Only human failure to find it, study and understand it, can diminish its value.[2]

Locard's Exchange Principle can be seen in all spheres of life: from the seashore to the African bushveld, from your eyelids and your bones to rhino horns, from forensic cases (such as the Unabomber case) to genocides, to your diet, to your accent, to the atom, to memes and to your relationships. Let me use these real-world examples to demonstrate Locard's Exchange Principle at work.

The seashore: A marine biologist can tell you what species exist in the ocean from the evidence washed up on the seashore. Given enough time, the marine biologist will have a relatively good idea of all the aquatic plants, fish, shellfish and bait organisms in a marine-protected area, without even venturing into the water of that area.

The African bushveld: A game-ranger can tell you if aardvark (antbear) (*Orycteropus afer*) or lion (*Panthera leo*) exist in a certain nature reserve without needing to see them, based solely on those species' contacts with the environment (footprints and dung).

Your eyelashes: *Demodex folliculorum*, a microscopic mite typically found on the skin and eyelashes of humans, is also transferred. Unbelievably, you and your partner share a demodex population! Demodex populations have been used to solve forensic cases.[3]

Bones: We can tell if skeletal remains date from before or after 1945. Pre-1945 skeletal bones are free of endogenous strontium-90 (a radioactive isotope of strontium produced by nuclear fission), derived from nuclear weapons and atmospheric tests, which were at a maximum in the environment in the early 1960s. Atmospheric contamination with isotopes laid down in skeletal bones from dated tests and nuclear accidents may therefore help date skeletal remains.[4]

Rhino horn: Locard's Exchange Principle could possibly help solve wildlife crime. By inserting measured quantities of radioisotopes into the horns of live rhinos, nuclear science might be able to assist with conservation. This non-lethal solution aims to reduce the demand from end-users and save rhinos from the threat of extinction. Making rhino horns radioactive reduces their desirability as a commodity. Radioactively treated horns are more likely to be detected at international borders, potentially exposing criminal syndicates and thereby ensuring that they are prosecuted and convicted under anti-terrorism laws. This science-based solution could help curb the demand for rhino horns and ultimately save a species. At its heart lies Locard's Exchange Principle.

The Unabomber: James R Fitzgerald, an American criminal profiler and retired FBI agent, used forensic linguistics (the application of linguistic knowledge, methods and insights to help investigate and solve crimes) in the arrest and conviction of Ted Kaczynski, the Unabomber. Fitzgerald studied the (initially anonymous) Unabomber's 35 000-word manifesto, and compared it to known documents from Kaczynski, which proved integral to solving the Unabomber case. Forensic linguistics adheres to Locard's Exchange Principle; Kaczynski had left traces of himself on all his documents.

Genocides: All genocides start in the same way. There is a recipe for genocides. This recipe adheres to Locard's

Exchange Principle. All genocides can be traced and tracked back to an original idea or ideology. There is typically an 'us and them' narrative. The ideology spreads its way throughout the society, via the media, through word of mouth, by means of Locard's Exchange Principle.

Your diet: You really are what you eat! At a glance, you can tell if a person is eating healthily or unhealthily. Traces of their diet can be seen in their skin, weight, mood and general well-being.

Your accent: Your accent is a distinctive way of pronouncing a language, especially associated with a particular country, area, or social class. Your accent is a classic example of Locard's Exchange Principle.

The atom: In 1911, Ernest Rutherford's gold foil experiment demonstrated that the atom had a tiny and heavy nucleus. He used alpha particles emitted by a radioactive element to expose the unseen world of atomic structure. Most of the beams went through the foil, but a few were deflected. Rutherford famously later said, 'It was almost as incredible as if you fired a 15-inch shell at a piece of tissue paper and it came back and hit you.'

A piece of gold foil was hit with alpha particles, which have a positive charge. Most alpha particles went right through. This showed that the gold atoms were mostly empty space. Some particles had their paths bent at large angles. A few even bounced backward. The only way this could have happened was if the atom had a small, heavy region of positive charge inside it. The Rutherford atomic model proved that the atom is mostly empty space, and most of the mass is in the nucleus, which is positively charged. If you think about it critically, this is nothing other than an application of Locard's Exchange Principle.

Memes, cultural and other: The term 'meme' (from the Greek *mimema*, meaning 'imitated') was introduced in 1976 by British evolutionary biologist Richard Dawkins in his work *The Selfish Gene*. By Dawkins' definition, memes are cultural ideas that spread and repeat themselves across society. A meme is therefore a unit of cultural information spread by imitation. Memes can also be images, videos or pieces of text, and so on, typically humorous in nature, that are copied and spread by internet users, often with slight variations. Memes are likable and are shared with a group. Everyone understands the intended message easily. The shareability of memes makes them popular in a cultural group, or even globally, because most people find them relatable. Memes obey Locard's Exchange Principle, in that they can be traced and tracked back to source.[5]

Relationships: Locard's Exchange Principle can help determine if your partner is cheating on you. You may find transferred make-up, perfume or aftershave on your partner, which may require an explanation. On the flip side, Locard's Exchange Principle may even save or spice up your relationship. Try, for example, recreating your partner's ideal evening when they get home from work. Locard's Exchange Principle will help keep you sharp and alert. If you become sufficiently expert at Locard's Exchange Principle you may even discover things about your partner which you originally did not know, thereby deepening your knowledge of them.

Epilogue

I want to propose a controversial idea: Can Locard's Exchange Principle make you a happier human being? And can it provide you with a better philosophy for growing older?

I have demonstrated to you just how pervasive Locard's Exchange Principle is and how it works. Forensic experts use it daily to catch really bad people. Now instead of applying it to crime, can you apply this forensic principle to your own life and to those around you? Can we use it to solve the unhappiness issue? Can we solve 'unhappiness' like we solve a crime scene?

Can the dead teach us to live happier lives? The dead, after all, have so much to teach the living. I believe that much of the unhappiness in this world is preventable. I also believe that an understanding of contact theory will help provide us with some kind of better philosophy for growing older.

They say you should know the limits of your responsibilities and abilities. I know I may be stepping out of my field of expertise, given that this is considered the realm of the psychiatrist, and many may wonder why I, as a forensic pathologist, offer advice about happiness and how best to grow old. In my defence, I would say that I end up reading far too many suicide notes – and yet I think these suicide notes represent very clear messages to the living, given their inherent wisdom. Therefore grant me this final chapter: I want to share what I have read and therefore what I have learned. (As mentioned, I am into pattern recognition, and over the past twenty years, I have detected a pattern in suicide notes.)

What can these teach us about human happiness? What can they teach us about growing older?

I have learned that there are often three main reasons why people take their own lives: relationship, work and health reasons. These are the three battlefronts of life.

Almost all human stressors can be slotted into one of these three battlefronts: your mother-in-law, your hay fever, your boss, your finances, material things, your environment, your underlying health, your underlying psychiatric conditions, your age, geography, public prejudices, your sex life, your gender, your identity, your feelings, your leisure, society, your religious or political beliefs, your clubs, and your leisure time – they all slot in. Sheehy called these the 'predictable crises of adult life'.[1]

I believe that Locard's Exchange Principle, applied with genuine and authentic sincerity, will positively impact your own life. By critically addressing these three main battlefronts, I believe, almost all human beings can be happier than they are right now. I also believe you will be equipped with a better philosophy for growing older.

The Relationship Battlefront

Sometimes, when I get someone lying on my autopsy table, the only thing that goes through my mind is: *'This person made some really bad choices in their life.'* For example, there may be signs of chronic drug or alcohol abuse. (This poor soul needed to be more discerning about whom they associated with in their life, and more discerning about their contacts in life.) If you hang out with the wrong kinds of people, surely they will infect you? The unhappy and the unlucky will likely infect you. And, if you are the cleverest person in the room, you are probably in the wrong room. Therefore find wiser people, happier people and healthier people than yourself. Infect yourself with them.

Beware of social isolation. Do not wall yourself off from life by living in your own mental vault and restricting yourself to the narrowest spheres of isolation. Open some of those windows and doors and escape from your own mental vault by allowing in new ideas. Most of your fears may well be born of fatigue and loneliness. Take stock of your own situation, and broaden your interests in other human beings and things. Relationships exist everywhere in life. Life is about your fellow man and your fellow woman. It is also about your relationship with yourself. However, if you live only for yourself, you are always in danger of being bored to death by repetition of your own views, thoughts and interests. Social isolation is dangerous.[2] Just as you can be infected by someone more positive or more negative than yourself, so too you too can infect those around you. Contact a friend you have not thought about in a long time.

Send a cheering message to someone sick, lonely or in pain. Be mindful of the overlooked minorities of society.

There are many people in this world who may be ghosted, fizzled, shunned, blocked, cut off and ignored. Try to forge relationships with the timid, the lonely, the shy, the forgotten and the wallflowers. Pick up your mobile phone and communicate with these isolated souls. However, on the other hand, be aware of your mobile phone and do not hide behind it. Arrange a real meeting, in real life, face to face. Instead of building a wall around yourself, build a bridge to other people. Light, food, water, life and love, the very things that can bring you happiness, cannot penetrate your high walls.

Encourage the discouraged: be of some service to your fellow human beings. Good deeds (and bad deeds) obey Locard's Exchange Principle. Most people are lonely and have no one to talk to. Your neighbour is most likely just as discouraged as you are, and people are often seeking a willing listener. A sympathetic listener is rare to find. You never realise how lonely you are until it's the end of the day and you have a bunch of things to talk about and no one to talk to. There is no human being who, if given the opportunity, does not like to have an audience, even if it consists of just one person.

When you listen to the discouraged, try not pin a label on them, and try not to hurl a sermon at them. Instead, try and summarise what they said, and see if they agree with your summary. If they do not agree, then try to summarise what they said again, and see if they agree with your new summary. Keep doing this until they agree. Only continue to speak once they have completely accepted your summary of what they have said. Once they have, ask them the following questions: 'What evidence would get you to change your mind?' and 'What would make you less discouraged?'

With Locard's Exchange Principle, it is possible to encourage the discouraged and energise the exhausted.[3]

Discipline: I heard someone say that children are just different these days. I disagree: children are the same. What has changed is a society that is now characterised by lowered expectations, a lack of discipline and an acceptance of disrespect. Manage what your children are exposed to. Remember Locard's Exchange Principle: every contact leaves a trace. Give kids boundaries, expectations, rules, limits, rewards and consequences. Teach them self-control and self-restraint. Teach them healthy lifestyles, and teach them discipline. They will rise to the challenge and exceed your expectations every time. Great empires are built on discipline.

Stop the ghosting and the fizzling: it is stupid to quarrel and have misunderstandings and useless to carry resentments and grudges throughout your life. 'Radio silence' is an immature way to resolve disagreements. Going 'dead air', slamming doors in people's faces, killing phone calls, and blocking and 'ghosting' people are childish behaviours (unless, of course, those people are really toxic, in which case please avoid them at all costs). Ask yourself if the relationship is worth saving or not. Ask yourself if it is healthy to continue with contact, or not. Decide accordingly.

Become more objective. Nature does not care about your private logic. Your private logic cannot be substituted for the unrelenting logic of generations of life and living. Nature never lies. The entertainment industry and films have tinkered with us. We have been exposed to some kind of social re-engineering. There are people who think that real love is a hand sliding down a window, like in the movie *Titanic*, or that real love is two people eating a single piece of spaghetti, like the movie *Lady and the Tramp*. The Hollywood version of love has entered our minds like worms entering peaches – via Locard's Exchange Principle. These ideas were shared with us like memes and we were influenced by them, persuaded by them, and proselytised by them. Mature love means real friendship – someone to share the joys and sorrows of life with. The most common injury I see in forensic pathology is a broken heart. How many crimes have been committed in the name of 'love'? I have seen countless deaths from love triangles (plus just a few from love rectangles, and fewer still from love tetra-hexa-flexagons).

The word 'love' should have its connotations changed. Do not retain childish or adolescent concepts of love. Try to become a better-adjusted, more mature adult, especially when it comes to your love relationships in life. Try to become more objective, more reasonable, more independent and more responsible.

Fact check: Read both conservative and radical newspapers, and learn to draw your own conclusions from the evidence that is presented to you by both. Beware of the narratives that are shared with you by the media. Know the difference between media and journalism. Journalism is the activity of *professionally* gathering, assessing, creating and presenting news and information, whereas 'media' simply describes the channel of communication. The media often sensationalise stories for commercial purposes. *The News* needs to make the news. In the past, TV had a 30-minute news bulletin; nowadays the news is on multiple channels continuously, 24/7, 365 days per year. Surely most of the content is not really news by the strictest definition of the term? What really upsets me is that murder does not make front-page headlines these days. To me, murder is news!

Everything is data. Everything is information. The question arises: what is important information and what is junk information? Can forensic techniques help us differentiate between important data and noise? Currently, there is so much information that it feels as if we are drinking from the fire hydrant of information. The cause of collective stupidity nowadays is not *too little* information, but *too much* information, and *too much* misinformation. We need to be logical, lucid and critical about what we come into contact with.

Ask yourself if your news source is reliable, credible and reputable. Spend only about thirty minutes a day on local news and international news. Don't disseminate your opinions, unless you have read widely on a subject.[4] It is easy to share false information, and untold damage can be caused by the dissemination of falsehoods. Ideas (and ideologies) are shared via Locard's Exchange Principle. Always fact-check your information. Once you understand the facts, try to cooperate to the best of your ability with the best standards of the social group in which you live.

The Work Battlefront

Beware of too much work. You need to take time to be with family and friends, because one day you may lift your head up and find that they are not there. While one may go through many personal sacrifices to become successful, one's personal life may be failing. Is there someone with whom you share your success? It is lonely at the top of the mountain and it is best to learn from other people's climbs. There is no glory in not taking a holiday.[5] Take time away. You will do more damage to yourself, your work and your relationships by not taking a break. Time away allows you to reflect, to think, to repair, to bond and heal. Do not neglect your other battlefronts.

Beware of too little work: Many forensic cases have their origin in boredom. While working hard and long hours may have a deleterious effect on some individuals, in my opinion not working at all – which inevitably results in boredom – is far more dangerous. As a species, we are all living longer.[6] How are we spending our extra years? The newly retired person probably spends the first three to six months of retirement pottering around their house. And yet, science and technology have given us a gift, which is actually a curse: more free time. If you are busy, there is little time to be troublesome. Being busy is probably one of the most important aspects of life, and work can be a source of salvation. Even if you are doing nothing, you must be *busy* doing nothing. The business of being busy is probably one of the most important aspects of life. The proverb 'Idle hands are the devil's playground' means that someone who is unoccupied and bored will be prey to mischief. Someone who has nothing to do will take part in something that will get them into trouble.

Some people can sit on their veranda the entire day, moving around with the sun. Other people can sit in a tavern or a coffee shop the entire day.

Earlier on I discussed the 'machine of the world'. When you were young, you were a consumer who did nothing to keep the machine of the world working. Eventually, you started working, and you became a cog in the wheel of the machine. When you retire, you are no longer part of the machine: you become a consumer once again. Help keep the machine of the world turning – it is an effective way to defeat boredom.

To be a better-adjusted human, you need to be socially useful. Make adequate use of your leisure time. I would suggest creative and artistic activities. Hobbies are an effective form of insurance against the boredom of old age. By helping others one also helps oneself, because that creates a sense of self-satisfaction.

How many books can you read, how many series can you watch, how many podcasts can you listen to and how much time can be spent on a hobby? Hobbies are not the complete solution to boredom: they are not enough on their own to stave off boredom. I would say, keep studying throughout life. Never stop reading and learning. For most of us, as soon as the degree or diploma is framed, education ceases. You cannot coast through life on the momentum of your school, college or university education. And just because you received a degree or a diploma does not make you an educated person. You have to keep abreast of an ever-changing world.

The battlefront of boredom needs to be attacked with Locard's Exchange Principle: share your knowledge. Do not be a literary or an intellectual miser, but rather infect others with your wisdom. Mentorship can also stave off boredom. Use your wisdom to teach others how the machine of the world works. And let others infect you with their wisdom. If you read, you will enjoy the companionship of some of the greatest minds whose writings you have studied.

The Health Battlefront

Your health encompasses your mental, spiritual and physical health. Know your risks. Know your family tree. Eat healthily. Drink healthily. Surround yourself with good people. Keep Locard's Exchange Principle in mind: each day, try to come in contact with something hopeful. Try to hear a stirring song, read a good book, see a fine picture or eat a good meal. Try to stimulate your senses. Sniff a scented flower. Try to speak to or visit a good friend. Whatever you do, be mindful of your contacts. Be attentive to yourself and to others. Some of your people may be feeling bombarded, stressed, pressured or overwhelmed. You have no idea what others are going through, just as they have no idea of your circumstances. People are just trying to survive and, as I have said, life is brutal. We are all here for each other until we die, so be kind. Let them come into *contact* with your kindness, and you should come into *contact* with theirs.

Forensic pathologists are very much aware of mental health issues. In our department, we have tea or coffee together every day at 09:30 and 15:30. Here we connect with one another and we talk. The tearoom is an excellent place to talk. A few nice words can really help. In fact, words may build people up or break people down, inspire or destroy, heal or reconcile. Words are the scalpels of language and so they should be chosen wisely. Words, too, are a form of contact.

Melancholia: Beware of dissatisfaction and restlessness, in yourself and others. I often look for discontent in the eyes of people, and when I notice it, I know something is afoot; I can sense that trouble is brewing. Dissatisfaction and restlessness obey Locard's Exchange Principle: they spread, infect and metastasise. The way to address dissatisfaction and restlessness is head-on. Ask if needs are not being met. Dissatisfaction and restlessness can lead to melancholia, which is a feeling of deep sadness. It may occur when you realise that you have thrown away the greater part of your life wasting time. The result: you become blue, deeply discouraged, or life-weary.

Focus on simple pleasures: Focus on simple pleasures in life, not pleasures that can hurt you. Base jumping, for example, is the recreational sport of jumping from fixed objects, using a parachute to descend safely to the ground. The name of the sport is derived from the acronym BASE, which stands for four categories of fixed objects from which one can jump: buildings, antennae (such as radio masts), spans (bridges) and earth (cliffs). If you meet base jumpers, you will be very taken by them. They are charming people, high on life itself. They may even persuade you to become a base jumper yourself. There is one problem with base jumpers, though: few have read the forensic pathology literature on base jumping. The lethal injuries in fatal base-jumping accidents result predominately from abrupt deceleration and blunt impacts.[7]

As you grow older try to enjoy the tranquil pleasures, not the wild ones, which can hurt you, because as you age, you are more likely to have accidents and more likely to fracture bones, which will take longer to heal.

The task of living: Spend your time on earth trying to solve earthly problems. Your existence needs to be attacked with insight and understanding. Don't waste your time trying to solve things which you don't have the tools to solve. Focus on solving your own problems and our collective problems here on earth right now. The more completely you understand your time on earth, the greater your courage to go on with the task of living. There are problems which you will never be able to solve. Thousands of men and women, far cleverer than ourselves, have tried to solve these problems over the centuries and have failed. Devote your time, attention, activities and interest to solving our own earthly problems right here, right now. Be objective. Do not defer your life. Help keep the machine of the world well lubricated and turning. Adopt a new centre of gravity, here in this real world. Be firm with your purpose and your decisions. Why aim for the moon and Mars, when you can spread your kindness and your wealth right here on earth, right now?

Old age: We grow old and we die. Senility and incontinence are what we have to look forward to in old-old age, yet these will not really be our problems – because we will be *incontinent* and *senile*! Our senility and incontinence will most likely become someone else's problem. Look the reality of old age in the face. Unlike the body, paradoxically, your spirit does not decay with the years; try to be philosophical about this fact. Try to grow old philosophically. Develop a stoic disregard for trifling matters. Do not torture your body in order to fool yourself that you are still young. Gracefully surrender the things of your youth.[8] Face-lifts, cosmetic surgery, flashy clothing, heavy drinking and social overactivity cannot dupe nature. In other words, beware of the 'forever young' movement. Nature never wanted us to be forever young. If it took you 15 minutes to walk across a small island when you were younger, take 30 minutes to walk across the same small island now that you are older. By slowing down your pace, you will enjoy the scenery more. Make the long reaches of your maturity interesting and peaceful. However, as you grow older, keep moving, keep exercising, keep stretching and know your risks.

'I regularly exercise. I do abdominal muscle and fall prevention exercises, and I walk around.'[9] This is the sage advice from one of my mentors, Dr Thomas Noguchi, who is still fit and strong well into his nineties (as mentioned earlier in this book).

The best insurance against melancholia, depression and a sense of futility in old age is the development of wide horizons and the cultivation of mental elasticity and interest in the world. Ask yourself what it is that you want, what constitutes a good day and what your goals are. Keep Locard's Exchange Principle in mind: be aware of your contacts as you grow older in life. Both positive and negative contacts leave their traces.

You probably want to wake up in the morning with a purpose. You probably want to open your refrigerator and find some pleasing food. You probably want a healthy environment with some pleasure, curiosity and play. You want to be busy, have good company (be it your own or that of another person, other people or a pet). Some wish to sit on a balcony or veranda soaking up the sunlight, while others prefer daily activities. Some want pleasant neighbours – or no neighbours – good infrastructure and education, regular access to electricity, water and waste removal, good transport, good schools, universities and technical universities, and reputable medical infrastructure. You probably want safe and scenic places to go on holiday, good care for the elderly and to be valued and appreciated. I am certain you want to live your life wholeheartedly. Most of all, you probably want minimal stress and a good night's sleep!

All the case studies in my book have demonstrated one golden thread: Locard's Exchange Principle.

Knowing this principle, I hope you come to this conclusion: your family, your friends, your culture, your subculture, your private life and your work have left their mark on you. Every book, every movie, every series, every podcast, every conversation has left its trace evidence on you. So too has every meal, snack, vitamin, news bulletin (conservative or radical), dose of medicine, Tik-Tok video, Tweet, YouTube video, advert, habit, pollen grain (your hay fever) . . . Everything. Every single thing!

Contact theory:
- You are the end result of all your contacts in life.
- All your contacts have left indelible traces on you.
- All your contacts have accumulated to make you who you are.
- All your contacts may have constrained who you could have become.

Therefore:
- Look objectively at your work, your health and your relationships.
- Ask who or what you came in contact with in your past.
- Ask who or what you are coming into contact with right now.
- Understand the consequences of your future contacts in life.
- Infect yourself with wiser, happier and healthier people and things.
- Use 'contact theory' to grow old healthily and philosophically (i.e. take care with your future contacts).

By doing so, you may become a wiser, healthier, happier human, you will grow old better – *and we forensic pathologists will have less work!*

Notes

PREFACE

1. Wander P, Iluyomade A, Sanmartin P, Gupta A, O'Sullivan M. 2016. 'A tell-tale handshake', in *Respiratory Medicine Case Reports*, 18:76–77. doi:10.1016/j.rmcr.2016.04.010.

CHAPTER 1 *Solving puzzles*

1. Simmons GT. 1992. 'Death by power car window: An unrecognized hazard', in *The American Journal of Forensic Medicine and Pathology* 13(2):112–114. doi:10.1097/00000433-199206000-00006.
2. Mills C. 2010. *This Too Will Pass*. Lynn East: Ithuthuko Investments.
3. Knight B. 1996. *Forensic Pathology*, second edition. London: Arnold Publishers, p. 1.

CHAPTER 2 *Locard's Exchange Principle*

1. Stauffer E. 2006. 'Dr Edmond Locard and trace evidence analysis in criminalistics in the early 1900s: How forensic sciences revolve around trace evidence', in *Proceedings of the American Academy of Forensic Sciences* X:81.
2. Smith S. 1959. *Mostly Murder*. London: Companion Book Club.

CHAPTER 4 *Via negativa*

1. Sapa. 2002. 'Adam and Eve get 20 years for murder'. IOL, 31 May. Available at https://www.iol.co.za/news/south-africa/adam-and-eve-get-20-yearsfor-murder-87488
2. Trumpeter A. 2015. 'What is the via negativa?' *Philosophyzer*, 8 April. Available at https://www.philosophyzer.com/via-negativa/
3. Hassan SH. 2021. 'Hassan: The case for via negative'. *Yale Daily News*, 5 May. Available at https://yaledailynews.com/blog/2021/05/05/hassan-thecase-for-via-negativa/
4. Robinson L, Makhoba AM, Bernitz H. 2020. 'Forensic case book: Mirror image "selfie" causes confusion', in *South African Dental Journal* 75(3):149–151. doi:10.17159/2519-0105/2020/v75no3a6.

5. Morris AG. 2011. *Missing & Murdered: A Personal Adventure in Forensic Anthropology*. Cape Town: Zebra Press, p. 52.

CHAPTER 5 *Making decisions with minimal data*

1. Flewett TH, Parker RG, Philip WM. 1969. 'Acute hepatitis due to Herpes simplex virus in an adult', in *Journal of Clinical Pathology* 22:60–66. doi: 10.1136/jcp.22.1.60.
2. Norvell JP, Blei AT, Jovanovic BD, Levitsky J. 2007. 'Herpes simplex virus hepatitis: An analysis of the published literature and institutional cases', in *Liver Transplantation* 13(10):1428–1434 doi:10.1002/lt.21250.
3. Ibid.
4. These include medication toxicity, such as acetaminophen, hypoperfusion states, viral haemorrhagic fever (yellow fever), disseminated intravascular coagulation, eclampsia, cytomegalovirus, adenovirus, herpes zoster virus and measles.
5. Payne-James J, Jones R. 2020. *Simpson's Forensic Medicine*, fourteenth edition. Boca Raton, FL: CRC Press.
6. Habbe D, Thomas GE, Gould J. 1989. 'Nine-gunshot suicide', in *The American Journal of Forensic Medicine and Pathology* 10(4):335–337. doi:10.1097/00000433-198912000-00012.
7. Payne-James, Jones, pp. 142–143.
8. Karlsson T. 1999. 'Multivariate analysis ("forensiometrics") – a new tool in forensic medicine: Differentiation between firearm-related homicides and suicides', in *Forensic Science International* 101(2):131–140. doi:10.1016/s0379-0738(99)00017-1.
9. Rosenthal JS. 2006. *Struck by Lightning: The Curious World of Probabilities*. Washington DC: Joseph Henry Press.
10. Saric N, Fabien L, Fischer J, Hermelin A, Massonnet G, Burnier C. 2021. 'A preliminary investigation of transfer of condom lubricants in the vaginal matrix', in *Forensic Science International* 325:110847. doi:10.1016/j.forsciint.2021.110847.
11. Smith S. 1959. *Mostly Murder*. London: Companion Book Club, p. 261.

CHAPTER 6 *Looking for clues*

1. Payne-James J, Busuttil A, Smock W. 2003. *Forensic Medicine: Clinical and Pathological Aspects*. London: Greenwich Medical Media.
2. See Suarez CA, Arango A, Lester JL III. 1977. 'Cocaine-condom ingestion: Surgical treatment', in *Journal of the American Medical Association* 238(13):1391–1392. doi:10.1001/jama.1977.03280140069024.
3. Rogers C. 2021.'"The scalpel is passed": A conversation with Dr Thomas T Noguchi', in *The American Journal of Forensic Medicine and Pathology*. 42(2):103–108. doi:10.1097/PAF.0000000000000659.

CHAPTER 7 *Almost everything leaves a trace*

1. Montanaro A. 1996. 'Formaldehyde in the workplace and in the home: Exploring its clinical toxicology', in *Laboratory Medicine* 27:752–758. Also,

Salkie ML. 1991. 'The prevalence of atopy and hypersensitivity to formaldehyde in pathologists', in *Archives of Pathology & Laboratory Medicine* 115:614–616.

2. Andrews JM, Sweeney ES, Grey TC, Wetzel T. 1989. 'The biohazard potential of cyanide poisoning during postmortem examination', in *Journal of Forensic Science*, 34:1280–1284, doi:10.1520/JFS12763J.

3. Andrews et al. 1989; Ludwig J. 1979. Current Methods of Autopsy Practice, second edition. Philadelphia: WB Saunders Co.; Baselt RC. 2000. 'Cyanide',in Baselt RC (ed). *Disposition of Toxic Drugs and Chemicals in Man*. Foster City, CA: Chemical Toxicology Institute, pp. 221–225.

4. Schwär TG, Loubser JD, Olivier JA. 1988. *The Forensic ABC in Medical Practice: A Practical Guide*. Pretoria: Haum Publishers, p. 277.

5. Ago M, Ago K, Ogata M. 2008. 'Two fatalities by hydrogen sulfide poisoning: Variation of pathological and toxicological findings', in *Legal Medicine* 10(3): 148–152. doi:10.1016/j.legalmed.2007.11.005; 2. Kage S, Takekawa K, Kurosaki K, Imamura T, Kudo K. 1997.'The usefulness of thiosulfate as an indicator of hydrogen sulfide poisoning: Three cases', in *International Journal of Legal Medicine* 110(4):220–222. doi:10.1007/s004140050071; Ballerino-Regan D, Longmire AW. 2010. 'Hydrogen sulfide exposure as a cause of sudden occupational death', in *Archives of Pathology & Laboratory Medicine*' 134(8):1105. doi:10.5858/2010-0123-LE.1; Tran TTM, Fiaud C, Sutter EMM, Villanova A 2003. 'The atmospheric corrosion of copper by hydrogen sulphide in underground conditions', *Corrosion Science* 45(12): 2787–2802. doi:10.1016/S0010-938X(03)00112-4.

6. Knight B. 1996. *Forensic Pathology*, second edition. London: Arnold Publishers, p. 352.

7. Madea B. 2014. *Handbook of Forensic Medicine*. Hoboken, NJ: Wiley Blackwell.

8. Kling GW, Evans WC, Tanyileke G, Kusakabe M, Ohba T, Yoshida Y, Hell JV. 2005. 'Degassing Lakes Nyos and Monoun: Defusing certain disaster', in *Proceedings of the National Academy of Sciences* 102(40):14185–14190. doi:10.1073/pnas.0502274102.

9. Saukko P, Knight, B. 2016. *Knight's Forensic Pathology*, fourth edition. Boca Raton, FL: CRC Press, p. 359.

10. Dunford JV, Lucas J, Vent N, Clark RF, Cantrell FL. 2009. 'Asphyxiation due to dry ice in a walk-in freezer', in *Journal of Emergency Medicine* 36(4): 353–356. doi:10.1016/j.jemermed.2008.02.051.

11. Saukko, Knight. 2016, p. 359.

CHAPTER 8 *Specific contacts leave specific traces*

1. Blumenthal R, Mabotja SS, Soul B. 2022. 'Double death electrocution in the bathtub', in *The American Journal of Forensic Medicine and Pathology* 43(4):e88–e92. doi:10.1097/PAF.0000000000000755.

2. Goiti IL, Urrutia HZ, Ríos JG, Arteta IL, Heras MS, Paniagua AS. 2019. 'Low voltage supervision systems: Technology, applications, use cases and deployment', paper 396 in *Proceedings of the 25th International Conference on Electricity Distribution*.

3. Staff reporter. 2010. 'Runaway train: Warning screams futile'. News24, 21 April. Available at https://www.news24.com/news24/runaway-train-warning-screams-futile-20100421

4. Andrews CJ, Reisner AD, Cooper MA. 2017. 'Post electrical or lightning injury syndrome: A proposal for an American Psychiatric Association's Diagnostic and Statistical Manual formulation with implications for treatment', in *Neural Regeneration Research* 12(9):1405–1412. doi:10.4103/1673-5374.215242.

5. Knight B. 1996. *Forensic Pathology*, second edition. London: Arnold Publishers, p. 322.

CHAPTER 9 *Cause and effect – did this cause that?*

1. Hanley B, Lucas SB, Youd E, Swift B, Osborn M. 2020. 'Autopsy in suspected COVID-19 cases', in *Journal of Clinical Pathology*. 73(5):239–242. doi.10.1136/jclinpath-2020-206522.

2. Heinrich F, Meißner K, Langenwalder F, Püschel K, Nörz D, Hoffmann A, Lütgehetmann M, Aepfelbacher M, Bibiza-Freiwald E, Pfefferle S, Heinemann A. 2021. 'Postmortem Stability of SARS-CoV-2 in Nasopharyngeal Mucosa' in *Emerging Infectious Diseases* 27(1):329–331. doi: 10.3201/eid2701.203112.

3. Papavarnavas N, Frankenfeld P, Singh P, Pickard H, Audley G, Jacobs A, Mbalo Q, Steinhaus N, Omar A, Maughan D. 2021. 'The best and worst of times: Effects of Covid-19 on junior doctors and medical students at GSH'. *SAMA Insider*, July, pp. 6–8.

4. Burton JL. 2003. 'Health and safety at necropsy', in *Journal of Clinical Pathology* 56(4):254–260. doi:10.1136/jcp.56.4.254.

5. Moreno C, Wykes T, Galderisi S, Nordentoft M, Crossley N, Jones N, et al. 2020. 'How mental health care should change as a consequence of the COVID-19 pandemic', in *The Lancet Psychiatry* 7(9):813–824. doi: 10.1016/S2215-0366(20)30307-2.

6. The so-called 'heads' or 'head product' is not to be confused with the so called 'angel's share', which is the amount of an alcoholic drink that is lost to evaporation when the liquid is being aged in porous oak barrels. Up to one per cent of the volume of the cask can be lost each year through evaporation.

7. Schwär TG, Loubser JD, Olivier JA. 1988. *The Forensic ABC in Medical Practice: A Practical Guide*. Pretoria: Haum Publishers.

8. Paul-Ehrlich-Institut. 2021. Report: 'Verdachtsfälle von Nebenwirkungen und Impfkomplikationen nach Impfung zum Schutz vor COVID-19 seit Beginn der Impfkampagne am 27.12.2020 bis zum 31.07 August. Available at https://www.pei.de/SharedDocs/Downloads/DE/newsroom/ dossiers/sicherheitsberichte/sicherheitsbericht-27-12-bis-31-07-21.pdf.

9. Bhullar MK, Gilson TP, Lee J. 2022. 'The public health role of medical examiner offices during COVID-19 and other mass fatality events', in *The American Journal of Forensic Medicine and Pathology* 43(2):101–104. doi: 10.1097/PAF.0000000000000749.

10. James C, Peterson DC. 2022. 'Spontaneous multiple arterial dissection in

a COVID-19-positive decedent', *The American Journal of Forensic Medicine and Pathology* 43(1):52–54. doi:10.1097/PAF.0000000000000737.

CHAPTER 10 *Look to the environment*

1. Morris S. 2018 'Python owner was killed by his 8ft-long pet, coroner rules'. *The Guardian*, 24 January. Available at https://www.theguardian.com/environment/2018/jan/24/python-owner-killed-8ft-long-coroner-dan-brandon

2. Bernitz H, Bernitz Z, Steenkamp G, Blumenthal R, Stols G. 2012. 'The individualisation of a dog bite mark: A case study highlighting the bite mark analysis, with emphasis on differences between dog and human bite marks', in *International Journal of Legal Medicine* 126(3):441–446. doi:10.1007/s00414-011-0575-4.

3. Ibid.

4. Jones S. 2001. *Almost Like a Whale: The Origin of Species Updated*. London: Black Swan.

5. Lauridson JR, Myers L. 1993. 'Evaluation of fatal dog bites: The view of the medical examiner and animal behaviorist', in *Journal of Forensic Sciences* 38(3):726–731. doi:10.1520/JFS13462J.

6. Robinson L, Bunn BK, Blumenthal R, Bernitz H. 2023. 'The "hypopigmented" bitemark: A clinical and histologic appraisal', in *International Journal of Legal Medicine* 137:99–104. doi:10.1007/s00414-022-02922-x.

7. Bernitz et al. 2012.

CHAPTER 11 *Weapons and Locard's Exchange Principle*

1. Zhang X, Cain MD, Williams CD, Spears TA, Poulos CK. 2021. 'G2 Research Radically Invasive Projectile: The importance of recognizing its imaging and autopsy patterns', in *The American Journal of Forensic Medicine and Pathology* 42(3):248–251. doi:10.1097/PAF.0000000000000669.

CHAPTER 12 *Why this, why now?*

1. Radiation control receives its regulatory mandate through the Hazardous Substances Act 15 of 1973, which classifies electronic generators of ionising radiation as Group III hazardous substances, and radioactive sources as Group IV hazardous substances.

2. Blumenthal R. 2023. 'Crowd control: Forensic pathological perspectives'. Presentation at 10th *African Society of Forensic Medicine International Conference*, Kigali, Rwanda, 7–10 March.

3. Koayashi M, Mellen PF. 2009. 'Rubber bullet injury: Case report with autopsy observation and literature review', in *The American Journal of Forensic Medicine and Pathology* 30(3):262–267. doi:10.1097/PAF.0b013e318187dfa8.

4. Smith S. 1959. *Mostly Murder*. London: Companion Book Club, p. 90.

5. Koayashi, Mellen. 2009.

6. Voiglio EJ, Fanton L, Caillot J-L, Neidhardt J-P H, Malicier, D. 1998. 'Suicide with "non-lethal" firearm', in Lancet 352(9131):882. doi:10.1016S0140-6736(05)60010-4.

7. Bettenhausen C. 2020. 'Tear gas and pepper spray: What protesters need to know'. *Chemical and Engineering News*, 18 June. Available at https://cen.acs.org/policy/chemical-weapons/Tear-gas-and-pepper-spray-What-protesters-need-to-know/98/web/2020/06

8. Steffee CH, Lantz PE, Flannagan LM, Thompson RL, Jason DR. 1995. 'Oleoresin capsicum (pepper) spray and "in-custody deaths"', in *The American Journal of Forensic Medicine and Pathology* 16(3):185–192. doi:10.1097/00000433-199509000-00001.

9. Browning N. 2012. "Israeli skunk" fouls West Bank protests'. Reuters, 3 September. Available at https://www.reuters.com/article/us-israel-palestiniansskunk-idUSBRE88208W20120903

10. Davies W. 2008. 'New Israeli weapon kicks up stink'. BBC News, 2 October. Available at http://news.bbc.co.uk/1/hi/world/middle_east/7646894.stm

11. Knell Y. 2015. 'Who, what, why: What is skunk water?' BBC News, 11 September. Available at https://www.bbc.com/news/magazine-34227609

12. Haar RJ, Iacopino V. 2016. Lethal in Disguise: *The Health Consequences of Crowd-Control Weapons*. PHR and INCLO. Available at https://www.inclo.net/pdf/lethal-in-disguise.pdf.

CHAPTER 13 *Rare and unusual cases*

1. Weyers CZ, Makhoba MA, Blumenthal R. 2022. 'Pulmonary aspiration of brain matter in a motor vehicle fatality: A case study', in *The American Journal of Forensic Medicine and Pathology* 44(1): e1–e3, doi:10.1097/PAF.0000000000000784.

2. Anthelmintics or antihelminthics are a group of antiparasitic drugs that expel parasitic worms (helminths) and other internal parasites from the body by either stunning or killing them and without causing significant damage to the host (https://en.wikipedia.org/wiki/Anthelmintic).

3. Blumenthal R, Hänert-van der Zee B. 2018. 'A fire extinguisher death: The Macklin effect', in *The American Journal of Forensic Medicine and Pathology* 39(2), 103–105. Doi:10.1097/PAF.0000000000000374.

4. Macklin CC. 1939. 'Transport of air along sheaths on pulmonic blood vessels from alveoli to mediastinum: Clinical implications', in *Archives of Internal Medicine* 64(5):913 –926. doi:10.1001/archinte.1939.00190050019003.

5. Johns Hopkins Medicine (n.d.) 'Pneumomediastinum'. Available at https://www.hopkinsmedicine.org/health/conditions-and-diseases/pneumomediastinum

6. The powder was composed of mono ammonium phosphate (34–94%), ammonium sulphate (1–58%), mica (<4%), magnesium aluminium silicate (1–30%), methyl hydrogen polysiloxane (<1%) and amorphous silica (<2%).

7. A polarisation microscope is a microscope that utilises polarised light to reveal detail in an object, used especially to study crystalline and fibrous structures.

8. Post-mortem cosmetic experts are skilled in reconstructing a body after autopsy; they are almost as skilled as plastic surgeons when it comes to suturing wounds. If the body is pale, they inject red dyes into the vessels

to create a less-pale look. If the body is jaundiced, they address the yellow colour with certain make-up. If post-mortem odour is an issue, they use special perfumes. (Embalming originated in Egypt, presumably in 3200 BC. Complex balms were used in recipes for pharaonic mummification. Some of these embalming recipes contained acyl lipids (fat/oil), conifer (pine) resin, aromatic plant extracts, a sugar/gum and natural petroleum. Jones J, Higham TFG, Chivall D, Bianucci R, Kay GL, Pallen MJ, Oldfield R, Ugliano F, Buckley SA. 2018. 'A pre-historic Egyptian mummy: Evidence for an 'embalming recipe' and the evolution of early formative funerary treatments', in *Journal of Archaeological Science* 100:191–200. doi:10.1016/j.jas.2018.07.011.)

9. Smith S. 1959. *Mostly Murder*. London: Companion Book Club.
10. Blumenthal R, Roth LB. 2021. 'Transdermal fentanyl death pact', in *The American Journal of Forensic Medicine and Pathology*: 43(2) e18–e20. doi: 10.1097/PAF.0000000000000732.

CHAPTER 14 *Occupational health and safety*

1. Hawkey PM, Pedler SJ, Southall PJ. 1980. 'Streptococcus pyogenes: A forgotten occupational hazard in the mortuary', in *British Medical Journal* 281(6247):1058. doi:10.1136/bmj.281.6247.1058.
2. Grist NR, Emslie J. 1985. 'Infections in British clinical laboratories, 1982–3', *Journal of Clinical Pathology* 38(7):721–725. doi:10.1136/jcp.38.7.721; Harrington JM, Oakes D. 1984. 'Mortality study of British pathologists 1974–80', in *Occupational and Environmental Medicine* 41:188–191. doi:10.1136/oem.41.2.188.
3. Pospisil L. 2000. 'A contribution to the history of glanders in the Czech Republic' in *Veterinární Medicína* 45(9):273–276.
4. Miller DC. 1988. 'Creutzfeldt-Jakob disease in histopathology technicians', *New England Journal of Medicine* 318:853–854. doi: 10.1056/NEJM198803313181312; Sitwell L, Lach B, Atack E, Atack D, Izukawa D. 1988 'Creutzfeldt-Jakob disease in histopathology technicians', *New England Journal of Medicine* 318:854; Brown P, Gibbs CJ, Gajdusek DC, Cathala F, LaBauge R. 1986. 'Transmission of Creutzfeld-JaKob disease from formalin-fixed, paraffin-embedded human brain tissue', *New England Journal of Medicine* 315:1614–1615. doi:10.1056/NEJM198612183152516.
5. Agent BZ (3-quinuclidinyl benzilate), for example, is an odourless, environmentally stable, white crystalline powder with anticholinergic activity. It is a psychotomimetic chemical warfare agent used as an anticholinergic hallucinogen.
6. Hanzlick R, Nolte K, deJong J. 2009. 'The medical examiner/coroner's guide for contaminated deceased body management', in *The American Journal of Forensic Medicine and Pathology* 30(4): 327–338. doi:10.1097/PAF.0b013e31819d208c.
7. Heptonstall J, Porter K, Gill ON. 1995. *Occupational Transmission of HIV*, summary of published reports, December. London: Public Health Laboratory Service, Communicable Disease Surveillance Centre.

8. Johnson MD, Schaffner W, Atkinson J, Pierce MA. 1997. 'Autopsy risk and acquisition of human immunodeficiency virus infection: A case report and reappraisal', in *Archives of Pathology & Laboratory Medicine*, 121(1): 64–66.
9. Burton JL. 2003. 'Health and safety at necropsy', in *Journal of Clinical Pathology* 56(4), 254–260. doi:10.1136/jcp.56.4.254, pp 254-260.

CHAPTER 15 *How to be a medical detective in your own life*

1. Aetiology: The study of the causes. For example, of a disorder. The word 'aetiology' is mainly used in medicine, where it is the science that deals with the causes or origin of disease, the factors which produce or predispose toward a certain disease or disorder (https://www.medicinenet.com/aetiology/definition.htm).
2. 'The dose makes the poison' is an adage intended to indicate a basic principle of toxicology. It is credited to Paracelsus, who expressed the classic toxicology maxim 'All things are poison, and nothing is without poison; the dosage alone makes it so a thing is not a poison.' This is often condensed to: 'The dose makes the poison.' or in Latin, '*Sola dosis facit venenum.*'

CHAPTER 16 *A recap of Locard's Exchange Principle*

1. Paul Leland Kirk 9 May 1902 – 5 June 1970 was a biochemist, criminalist and participant in the Manhattan Project. Kirk was an avid supporter of Locard's Exchange Principle. He said that the real aim of all forensic science was to establish 'individuality'. Criminalistics is the science of individualisation.
2. Kirk PL. 1953. Crime Investigation: *Physical Evidence and the Police Laboratory*. New York: Interscience Publishers.
3. Ozdemir MH, Aksoy U, Akisu C, Sönmez E, Cakmak MA. 2003. 'Investigating demodex in forensic autopsy cases', in *Forensic Science International* 135(3): 226–231. doi: 10.1016/s0379-0738(03)00216-0.
4. Maclaughlin-Black S M, Herd R J, Willson K, Myers M, West IE. 1992. 'Strontium-90 as an indicator of time since death: A pilot investigation', in *Forensic Science International* 57(1):51–56. doi:10.1016/0379-0738(92)90045-x.
5. Dawkins R. 1990. *The Selfish Gene*, second edition. Oxford: Oxford University Press.

EPILOGUE

1. Sheehy G. 1977. *Passages: Predictable Crises of Adult Life*. New York: Bantam.
2. If you are forced to live in social isolation, then you need a proper management plan. Surviving solitary confinement is an art and a science.
3. Wolfe WB. 1937. *How to be Happy Though Human*. London: George Routledge & Sons.
4. Brown D. 2017. *Happy: Why More or Less Everything is Absolutely Fine*, first printing edition. Whitman.

5. Kubheka M. 2016. *Vuyo's: From a Big Big Dreamer to Living the Dream.* Johannesburg: Tracey McDonald Publishers.
6. Roser M, Ortiz-Ospina E, Ritchie H. 2019. 'Life expectancy', *Our World in Data.* Available at https://ourworldindata.org/life-expectancy.
7. Wolf BC, Harding, BE. 2008. 'Patterns of injury in a fatal BASE jumping accident', in *The American Journal of Forensic Medicine and Pathology* 29(4):349–351. doi:10.1097/PAF.0b013e318184fb12.
8. Ehrmann M. 1948. 'Desiderata', in Ehrmann BK (ed.) *The Poems of Max Ehrmann.* Boston: Bruce Humphries Inc.
9. Rogers C. 2021.'"The scalpel is passed": A conversation with Dr Thomas T Noguchi', in *The American Journal of Forensic Medicine and Pathology.* 42(2):103–108. doi:10.1097/PAF.0000000000000659.

Glossary

Asphyxiation: The state or process of being deprived of oxygen, which can result in unconsciousness or death; suffocation.

Creutzfeldt–Jakob disease (CJD), also known as subacute spongiform encephalopathy or neurocognitive disorder due to prion disease, is an invariably fatal degenerative brain disorder.

Encephalopathy: Damage or disease that affects the brain.

Glanders: An infectious disease that is caused by the bacterium *Burkholderia mallei.* While people can get the disease, glanders is primarily a disease affecting horses. It also affects donkeys and mules and can be naturally contracted by other mammals such as goats, dogs and cats.

Globus pallidus: The median part of the lentiform nucleus in the brain.

Inotropic support: Inotropic agents, or inotropes, are medicines that change the force of your heart's contractions. There are two kinds of inotropes: positive inotropes and negative inotropes. Positive inotropes strengthen the force of the heartbeat. Negative inotropes weaken the force of the heartbeat.

Immunocompromised: When you are immunocompromised, your immune system's defences are low, affecting its ability to fight off infections and diseases. Depending on why your immune system is compromised, this state can be either permanent or temporary.

Immunohistochemistry: A laboratory method that uses antibodies to check for certain antigens (markers) in a sample of tissue. The antibodies are usually linked to an enzyme or a fluorescent dye. After the antibodies bind to the antigen in the tissue sample, the enzyme or dye is activated, and the antigen can then be seen under a microscope. Immunohistochemistry is used to help diagnose diseases such as cancer. It may also be used to help tell the difference between different types of cancer.

Lines of Zahn: A characteristic of thrombi that appear particularly when formed in the heart or aorta. They have visible and microscopic alternating layers (laminations) of platelets mixed with fibrin, which appear lighter, and darker layers of red blood cells.

Linguistics: The scientific study of language and its structure, including the study of grammar, syntax and phonetics. Specific branches of linguistics include sociolinguistics, dialectology, psycholinguistics, computational linguistics, comparative linguistics and structural linguistics.

Necrosis: The death of most or all the cells in an organ or tissue due to disease, injury or the failure of the blood supply.

Polarisation: The attribute of a wave referring to its oscillations in a definite direction relative to the direction of propagation of the wave.

Post hoc, ergo propter hoc: Latin for '*After this, therefore because of this*', which is a logical fallacy (of the questionable cause variety) postulating that since event B *followed* event A, event B must have been *caused* by event A. It is often shortened to *post hoc* and is sometimes referred to as false cause, coincidental correlation, or correlation not causation.

Pulmonary embolism: This occurs when a clump of material, most often a blood clot, gets wedged into an artery in your lungs.

Streptococcus: A bacterium of which there are several types. Two of them cause most of the strep infections in people: group A and group B. A strep throat refers to a sore, red throat.

Acknowledgements

Countless ideas derived from the works of other writers have been incorporated into this book. The cases cited in the text have been drawn from my own forensic case files. Most have been published and have been through the peer-review process. In other cases, names, dates and places, together with all personal data which could lead to the identification of the individuals, have been altered to preclude all possibility of reasonable recognition.

I would like to express my deepest gratitude to all those who, knowingly or unknowingly, added to this book, and to all those who keep the machine of this world turning.

My sincerest gratitude to my publisher, Annie Olivier, and editor, Carol-Ann Davids, and to all the staff at Jonathan Ball Publishers. Thanks to Eugene Ashton for inspiring this journey.

Special thanks to my parents, Walter and Diane, for their unwavering support.

Thanks to my brother, Darren, for his wonderful and positive attitude.

Thanks to my uncle Brian Blumenthal for his sound legal advice.

Thanks to my uncle Julius Preddy for his kind support and friendship.

Thanks to my legal advisor, Annelize Nienaber and my colleagues who proofread this manuscript.

Thanks to those who have helped me develop my understanding of 'contact theory' over the years.

Finally, to my forensic colleagues in South Africa and abroad – thank you.